Reflections
from COMMON GROUND...
Cultural Awareness in Healthcare

Beth Lincoln, MSN, RN

with narratives by Cody Gillette Kirkham

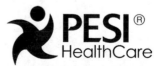

PESI®
HealthCare

EAU CLAIRE, WISCONSIN
2010

D0089448

For information on this and other
PESI HealthCare products
please call 800-843-7763 or
visit our website at www.pesihealthcare.com

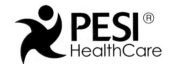

Cover Graphic by Jon Dodge

Peer Reviews

In REFLECTIONS from COMMON GROUND: Cultural Awareness in Healthcare, author and transcultural nurse Beth Lincoln captures the essence of cultural competency. The book encourages readers to reflect on culture, their own and those of others, and motivates them to begin their journeys toward culturally competent care. It puts culture in an historical context and encourages healthcare providers to view themselves and their patients within that cultural framework. Because of the continuous increase in diversity in this country, healthcare providers should read and use this book to bridge the gap between culture and care, and help eliminate healthcare disparities.

Lorraine Steefel, DNP, RN, CTN-A, Certified Transcultural Nurse,
Member of the Transcultural Nurses Society,
National Speaker on Issues related to Cultural Competency/Diversity, Professional
Writer/Writing Consultant,
Adjunct Assistant Professor UMDNJ School of Nursing, Newark, NJ.

Reflections from Common Ground offers a rich and insightful exploration into the perceptions of the past and our sensitivities in the present. Beth Lincoln has created an anthology of cultural experience for us to explore, contemplate and from which to grow. Fascinating! A valuable tool for all of us ~

Jennifer Kresge MFCC, Healthcare Mediator & National Speaker

Dedication . . . To those who paved the way

Dr. Madeleine Leininger ~ Culture Care Theorist
Culture Care Diversity and Universality

Dr. Rachel Spector
Cultural Diversity in Health and Illness

Dr. Larry Purnell
Transcultural Health Care: A Culturally Competent Approach

Drs Joyce Giger and Ruth Davidhizer
Transcultural Nursing: Assessment and Intervention

Drs Margaret Andrews and Joyceen Boyles
Transcultural Concepts in Nursing Care

Dr. Josepha Campinha-Bacote
The Process of Cultural Competence in the Delivery of
Healthcare Services

Drs Juliene Lipson, Suzanne Dibble & Pamela Minarik
Culture & Nursing Care: A Pocket Guide

Acknowledgements

Find your voice!
Nancy Felling

Ma . . . you gotta write a book!
Son ~ Rudy McClain

Even when . . . it's all good
Son ~ Malcolm McClain

It doesn't surprise me . . .I knew you could do it!
Cindy Matheny

Oh, the stories she can tell . . .
Cody Gillette Kirkham

What's the book about. . .11th hour title change
Jennifer Kresge

Certified to find common ground in the midst of diversity
Lorraine Steefel, Magie Conrad & Betty Klecker

Editing . . . Editing . . . Editing . . . and then some
Nancy Felling, Jan Darter, Cody Gillette Kirkham

Tuesday Women's Group . . . the Wise & Wonderful
Nancy Garden, Ruthie Rydman, Jackie Gumina, Anne Anderson,
Lois Swanson, Cody Kirkham, Nancy Felling,
Cathy Marsten, Sue Fish & Susan French

Always there . . . Always supportive – the sibs
Ann, Bill, Dee, Mary, Barby, John, Jim, David & Lynn Lincoln

The Art of being and doing!
Hubby ~ aka Jon Dodge

Honored and proud daughter of
Barbara and Bill Lincoln

. . . HOW COME NO ONE EVER TOLD ME

ALL THROUGHOUT HISTORY

THE LONELIEST PEOPLE

WERE THE ONES WHO ALWAYS SPOKE THEIR TRUTH

THE ONES WHO MADE A DIFFERENCE

WITHSTANDING INDIFFERENCE

I GUESS IT'S UP TO ME NOW

SHOULD I TAKE THE RISK

OR SHOULD I JUST SMILE . . .

- THE KINGS OF CONVENIENCE

Oye, E., Boe, E., (June, 2004)
Album: Riots in an Empty Street
Song: Misread
Label: Astrawerks
Producer: Kings of Convenience

Table of Contents

The Journey . . .
A Conscious
Decision

1

Our world is changing, the demographics of our country are changing and we, as healthcare providers (HCPs), are asked to deliver care that "fits with and is useful to the client and family," according to Dr. Madeleine Leininger (1991 p. 39), Culture Care Theorist. The impetus of this book, for me, was the voices of patients encountered on my journey, especially those whose ethnicity and culture were different from mine. They were saying, "You need to tell our stories." The result – *Reflections from Common Ground*.

This book is an opportunity for you to engage in self-reflective exercises, to discover your culture and to realize how your culture influences every encounter. With each activity you'll discover something unique about yourself. Your ways of living in the world, your style of communication, your approach to health and illness, and therefore your response to a given situation are dictated by your culture. Each insight enables you to understand your differences with other people and to find common ground.

Reflections from Common Ground addresses the challenges and celebrates the accomplishments of providing culturally sensitive and competent healthcare. It is not a "cookbook" approach on how to deliver healthcare to diverse populations. A checklist is not included. Why? Because, in reality, there is more diversity within a cultural group than between groups. A recently arrived Mexican immigrant is going to be different from a fourth generation Mexican American. The African American whose history is rooted in slavery is different from the newly arrived immigrant from countries in Africa today. It is helpful for HCPs to learn about the patient's history – their story – before making assumptions based on ethnicity. How you manage the complexity of a situation to address patient's needs is contingent on knowledge of the cultural values, beliefs, and health practices of various ethnic groups.

1

The vignettes, found in chapters ten through twenty, are a compilation of experiences written in a fictional format. The purpose of the stories is to bring to life events that challenge the HCP to provide care that addresses culture and its influence on decisions about healthcare, from the pregnant Mexican American woman (Chapter Ten) to the elderly Hmong gentleman (Chapter 17) who presents in the emergency room with gastrointestinal bleeding, to the youth-oriented Anglo American woman (Chapter 20) with hypertension. Each will pique your interest and desire to know more. The vignettes are not meant to stereotype, but rather to highlight each aspect of particular cultures. Although Monica McGoldrick's book *Ethnicity and Family Therapy* is in its third edition she said it well in the introduction of her second edition. "Although stereotyping or generalizing about groups has often reinforced prejudices, one cannot discuss ethnic cultures without such generalizing. The only alternative is to ignore this level of analyses of group patterns which in our view only mystifies and disqualifies our experience thus perpetuating covert negative stereotyping only if allowed to air assumptions we can learn about each others' ethnicity" (p 22).

The vignettes offer insight into another world. They highlight cultural values, beliefs, and healthcare practices. You discover in this process the similarities and differences between your culture and that of the individual in the story. As a HCP, you have the opportunity to incorporate both perspectives, yours and your patient's, into a plan of care. Positive health outcomes are more likely when differences are recognized and collaboration with the patient and family is utilized.

Setting the Stage

"Setting the stage" is a phrase used with many cultural groups and with actors! It refers to setting aside time at the beginning of an event, an appointment or a presentation to get things in order. It may involve socialization – chatting with colleagues from the previous shift or with a patient – before focusing on the reason for the appointment. The first nine chapters of this book set the stage. Chapters Two and Three focus on demographics and history – the stories behind the individual – and their influence on health decisions. Reflective exercises guide you to discover your own story. How is it the same or different from others? Answers lead to the acknowledgment that individual biases can stem from historical events and can lead to prejudice and discrimination (Chapter 4), thus furthering disparities in care. It is interesting to see the correlation of history with current health issues found in various ethnic groups today.

Chapters Five and Six highlight other obstacles that continue to affect health outcomes. We must be aware of each. For example, in the United States, thirty seven million persons live in poverty, fifty percent of African American and Latino youth drop out of high school before graduation, and nearly 14 million Americans are not proficient in English. The National Assessment of Adult Literacy (2006) found that eight million persons cannot read the label *"keep out of reach of children."* It's important to note that barriers such as income, education, language, and literacy play a role in the delivery of care. You are the link between the patient and care. You can bridge the gap and provide information the patient needs to restore health and well-being.

Culturally sensitive and competent care, discussed in Chapters Seven and Eight, is the foundation needed to care for diverse populations. It begins with HCPs' desire to know more about themselves and to respect and value their culture. It is followed by a motivation to learn about others. How are my cultural ways of living and working similar to or different from my patient's? How do I define health and illness? What treatment methods do I consider most effective? Chapter Nine, *Ancient Wisdom . . . Modern Medicine*, explores various healing methods and brings an awareness that there is a varied approach to healing. The best way to acknowledge these beliefs is to incorporate the beneficial practices into the patient's plan of care.

Each of these "setting the stage" chapters affords you the opportunity to discover the richness of your culture and your interactions with others. This self-reflective process enables you to understand culture and to communicate with your patients and colleagues in an effective and respectful manner.

A Variety of Approaches . . . You Choose

Variety is a hallmark of *Reflections from Common Ground*. This book provides multiple approaches that healthcare organizations (Chapter 22), health occupation faculty (Chapter 23), and individuals can use to gain cultural awareness and competence.

An organization or hospital may want to use the information in this book to ensure a culturally competent staff that also meets criteria for Joint Accreditation Commission of Health Care Organizations (JACHO), Magnet Status Recognition, or the Office of Minority Health's Culturally and Linguistically Appropriate Standards. It is important to demonstrate that staff members have attended required diversity programs and show that they are knowledgeable about the cultural values, beliefs, and practices of various ethnic populations.

Health occupation faculty can use the book to achieve multiple goals: meet accreditation requirements, gain cultural awareness and competence for faculty, or provide an adjunct textbook for students.

Prior to beginning the process of becoming more culturally aware, it is recommended to hold staff meetings to discuss the proposal. To be an effective program, staff/faculty must have an opportunity to review the subject matter, ask questions, raise objections, and make recommendations. It is important that they, as a group, demonstrate a willingness to participate, and agree to set time aside for this process. The program should be evaluated at intervals and revised as needed.

As an individual, you may recognize an inner readiness and desire to delve into the cultural world of the "other." It is in this process that you discover yourself, your beliefs, your values, and your practices. Those "aha moments" open you to unexpected revelations that change your perspective. You begin to see the world through the "eyes of the other." This new outlook sends a message to your clients, patients, and colleagues that you acknowledge there may be differences, but that you are open to finding common ground. This new understanding enables you to develop trusting and respectful relationships.

Reflections from Common Ground provides a venue for you, the HCP, to recognize the significance and value of culture and its influence on health practices and decisions, and to supply the knowledge and skills needed to provide culturally sensitive, competent, and respectful care. Enjoy the journey . . .

History . . .
It Influences
Us Every Day

2

And it began . . .

Reflective exercise: Your story
1. *When did your ancestors first come to America?*
2. *Or were they already here?*
3. *Why did they come?*
4. *Share your story:*

Speaking in his native Pomo language, a recent conference speaker explained that his grandfather had told him "Your life is your story . . . tell your story." Whatever our native language, we all have a story to tell; in sharing our story, we gain insights into our history and those who came before us. Our histories, our stories, shape who we are and influence how we see and interpret our world.

Recently, a young woman shared that she had fled Cambodia, and spent four years in a refugee camp in Thailand before immigrating to the United States. Her colleagues never knew that piece of her history. It now provides a perspective, a way of seeing her with new understanding. Now transfer this process to your patients and colleagues. How are their stories similar to yours? How are they different?

In this chapter we will look at history and the effect it may have on healthcare decisions. For some the reason to seek, or not seek, healthcare may be based on previous encounters by family members or a long-standing history of mistrust of the system. Although these incidents may have happened many years in the past, it is in sharing of stories that one formulates beliefs, values, and biases about healthcare and healthcare providers.

Our story begins . . .

. . . with those who were here in America before the emigration from Europe and Asia. It begins with a Pequot man, standing on the shore of the Atlantic Ocean, watching the first white settlers arrive in this, his country. Until that time, there were, according to Charles Mann (2005), author of *1491: New Revelations about Americas before Columbus*, over 90 million Indians living on 400 million acres. Their advanced level of farming and hunting and gathering had sustained them over thousands of years. It was a thriving community of peoples across the Americas – North and South. The first of many treaties with the Native American population began in the early 1800s when then Major General Andrew Jackson defeated the Creeks in what is now the state of Alabama. Over twenty million acres of tribal land were seized in the 1814 treaty. The desire by Americans to establish a solid economic base, along with their disregard for the native people currently inhabiting the land, continued this process for the next one hundred years.

Economics always seems to be at the forefront of immigration to the Americas. The early 17th century saw increased emigration from England – people seeking a better life for themselves and their families. The 1700s and 1800s brought immigrants all seeking work with the ability to send money home. They came from Italy, Germany, Ireland, Asia, and South America. For many, the intent was to return to their homeland, but less than half realized that dream. Other emigrations stemmed from wars, famines, and reunification. Forced immigration (slavery) added to the socioeconomic status of the plantation owner, but did nothing for that of the slave. Forced migration, the movement of people to a land inconsistent with their lifestyle, affected most of the Native Americans who had not already been killed by guns or germs. Immigration by white settlers, unfortunately, brought disharmony and distrust.

Troubled Times Lead to Emigration

England

Following King Henry VIII's establishment of the Anglican Church, Protestants and Catholics alike were subject to shunning by neighbors, and were also fined and occasionally jailed by the government. Some Protestants took the Reformation as an opportunity to go one step further and "purify" the Anglican Church. They called themselves Puritans and believed that they did not need an intermediary (priest), but that they could talk to God on their own. This created a religious tumult in England. The

North American colonies probably seemed like an answer to prayer: the possibility of religious freedom. In 1620 the Pilgrims, as they came to be known, sailed on the Mayflower for the new colonies.

The 17th century focused on the establishment of colonies. During this time the economy in England was unstable, and inflation led to poverty, making it next to impossible for the poor to meet even their basic needs. For many the opportunity to leave for the new colonies was the answer. By the mid-1600s, more than 30,000 people had left for the new colonies. King James I viewed this as a win-win for England: an outlet for surplus population and input of material for their expansive industry.

As time went on, there was a greater sense of establishment in this new country with a growing desire to separate from England's rule. What followed was the Declaration of Independence in 1776. It is interesting to note that it was not until 1787 that the term immigrant was used. The term differentiated between the colonists who saw themselves as the established society and those *foreigners* who arrived after the country's laws, customs, language, and constitution were formed. This may have been done in response to Thomas Malthus' published *Essay on Principles of Population* in 1789. It stated that England was quickly running out of food production and predicted that if nothing changed starvation would result. A surge of immigrants to America followed. Wars and famine were another reason for migration.

China

In China the Opium Wars involving England (1836) and France (1846) created a very difficult situation. Because the wars decimated the land, agriculture was slow to recover and famine was the order of the day. Since there was not enough food to sustain families, many Chinese emigrated to America to work on the railroads, in the gold mines, in agriculture, and in factories. Sending money home and repaying the merchant who had brought them to the United States forced them to work at low wages. While many Chinese were successful and thrived, residents of the United States saw this as a threat to their livelihood. Chinese communities formed as a source of support, but stories of prostitution, gambling, and opium dens sparked the sentiment that admitting Chinese into the United States lowered the cultural and moral standards of American society (U.S. Department of State). Anti-Chinese sentiment rose and pursuant to a downturn in the economy, legislation was passed to bar immigration from China. That 1882 law, known as The Chinese Exclusion Act, was renewed in 1892 and again in 1902. It was not repealed until 1943.

Ireland

Poor economic conditions and famine played a key role in the Irish coming to America as well. Farmers in Ireland rarely owned the land, but rather rented it from landowners living in England. The cost of running the farm, however, left little money with which to support themselves and their families. Emigration to America began in the early 1800's and escalated following the potato famines of 1845 and 1846. One-fourth of the population emigrated to the United States. On a recent trip to Ireland our tour guide, Sean O'Malley, shared his family history with us. "The only time I ever heard my great grandfather talk about the great famine was during a family celebration. He recalled the people who left. It was the thought at that time that when someone left they would never be mentioned again. It was as if they had died." You could hear the sadness in Sean's voice as he told his story.

Italy and Germany

With increased taxation and low wages in Italy in 1870, many people emigrated to the United States. The intention was to make money and then return home. Many were not able to fulfill their dream; however, emigration to the U.S. continued from many European countries. It is noted that between 1820 and 1920, 4,400,000 immigrated from Ireland, 5,500,000 from Germany, and 4,190,000 from Italy. Most came for the same reasons: looking for economic stability and a better life for themselves and their families (Brunner 1997).

Mexico

Following the Mexican American war of 1848, those living in the southwestern area of the country, which was ceded to the United States by Mexico, were given U.S. citizenship with all the rights and privileges of others already living in the states. The Treaty of Guadalupe Hidalgo promised citizenship, freedom of religion and language, and maintenance of their lands. The Mexicans who lived in the southwest were subject to discrimination and social injustice following the war. Loss of both property and rights followed as well (McGoldrick 2005). Socioeconomic stability and labor needs have continued to play an integral part in the migration from Mexico to the United States. Borders, being permeable and allowing for flow back and forth, met the needs of both countries. In the mid-1800s, laborers were provided by Mexico to work on the railroad and in agriculture, thus proving a source of income for the Mexicans and a source of revenue for their country. This win-win relationship continued into the early 1900s, until there was a sudden downturn in the economy: the Great Depression. All immigration was stopped. It was not until there was a labor shortage during World War II that the borders reopened. The Bracero program, instituted in 1942 by the United States and Mexican governments, provided Mexican men to work in U.S. fields for low wages. The Bracero program caused resentment with the farm workers. Cesar Chavez initiated the Farm Workers Union to support those working in agriculture with just wages and living conditions. The Bracero Program ended in 1964 due to pressure from the union.

The needs of individuals, regardless of their countries of origin, played a significant role in the search for stability and economic security for themselves and their families. When there is a socioeconomic downturn, there may be a perception that immigrants are taking away jobs by working for low wages. The facts do not always back up that notion. Yet when there is a threat to economic wellbeing, fear, anger, and uncertainty loom.

Forced Immigration . . . Slavery

Economics. The reasons for slavery may have been many, but the bottom line was economic. Slaves were laborers who were owned: laborers who were told what to do, laborers who were told how to live. African slaves in the U.S. prior to 1865 had no rights and were considered less than whole people. They were counted as 3/5 of a person in the census report (U.S. Constitution, 1787). It is said that between three and twenty-four million slaves were brought to the United States. It does remain a fact that slavery existed for over three hundred years in this country. Families were separated. Men, women, and children were bought and sold. Living conditions were well below standard. Treatment of, and punishment for, perceived "crimes" was harsh. Slavery is a part of our story: it continues to influence us.

Not until the conclusion of the U.S. Civil war was slavery abolished. The passage of the 13th, 14th, and 15th amendments abolished slavery and established the right of citizenship, which included the right to own land and serve on a jury. Unfortunately, "Jim Crowe" laws, anti-African legislation passed after the Civil War, followed these constitutional amendments, continuing to affect the former slaves' ability to realize their constitutional rights. It would be years later with the passage of the 1964 Civil Rights Act and the 1965 Voting Rights Act that the laws established one hundred years earlier would actually take effect and become reality.

9

Forced Migration . . . and its effects

The recent PBS documentary, *Our National Parks* (2009), emphasized that much of the land in parks such as Yosemite, Yellowstone, Zion, and the Grand Canyon had been home to the native population for thousands of years. Displacement of Native Americans through forced migration from the "familiar" to unfamiliar land (which came to be known as reservations) changed their way of life. *The Indian Removal Act of 1830* authorized the federal government to negotiate treaties with Indian nations, exchanging their land for land in the West. After treaties had been signed some of the Indians left while others remained. In 1827, the Cherokee Nation adopted a written constitution declaring itself a sovereign nation legally capable of ceding its own land. The state of Georgia (where they resided) did not recognize that sovereignty. In 1831 the Cherokee nation took its case to the Supreme Court, and while winning the appeal initially, had its decision revoked later. Forced migration occurred throughout the 1830s from the *Trail of Tears* of the Cherokee Nation to Oklahoma, to "forced march" of the Piautes from Owens Valley to Fort Tehan in California. In each case thousands of persons perished due to lack of food, disease, and harsh conditions. Millions of acres were lost, but more than that, lost was the land that had been home for hundreds of years.

The Bureau of Indian Affairs formed in 1824. Responsible for the management of millions of acres of land "held in trust by the United States for the American Indians," the Bureau provided Indian health and social services in exchange for the land and natural resources. In 1978 Public Law 95-341 was enacted. The law stated "it shall be the policy of the United States to protect and preserve for American Indians their inherent right of freedom to believe, express and exercise the traditional religions of the American Indian, Eskimo, Aleut and Native Hawaiian, including but not limited to access to sites, use and possession of sacred objects and the freedom to worship through ceremonials and traditional sites" (U.S. Department of the Interior). Prior to this, American Indians did not have access to a number of sacred sites situated on federal lands such as national parks.

Another attempt to change the life of the Native American was the formation of the Carlisle Indian Schools in 1879. Started by Richard Henry Pratt, whose adage was "kill the Indian, save the man," the schools ensured that children who attended were prohibited from speaking their tribal language or wearing any clothing that was reflective of their nation. The goal was to forcibly assimilate Native American children into majority American culture. Yet it was not until 1924 that American Indians became citizens of the United States.

Ellis Island and Immigration

There were more than thirty seven million immigrants who passed through Ellis Island between 1892 and 1954, when it closed. Immigrants came for a variety of reasons, including political and economic stability, religious freedom, and family reunification. During World War I, Ellis Island was used as a site for suspected enemy aliens who were then transferred to other facilities. In the 1920s, public sentiment and politicians were beginning to voice concerns over the increased number of immigrants entering the United States. Restrictive laws, similar to The Chinese Exclusion Act and The Alien Contract Labor Law, along with the initiation of a literacy test, helped to deter the aspiring newcomers. The 1924 the National Origins Act limited the number of immigrants each year to two percent of any current ethnic group. The largest number of the immigrant spots were allocated to those coming from Northern and Western Europe, the least from Southern and Eastern Europe. The Act prohibited those entering from Asia altogether. Due to the current labor shortage, there was no restriction for Mexico (U.S. Department of the Interior).

So why bring up past events that now appear resolved?

History, one's story, may influence decisions about seeking healthcare – trust and relationship being key issues. These histories had an impact on health outcomes. Read on.

Recent History . . .

<u>Reflective Exercise</u>: **Were you or your parents or grandparents alive when . . .**

1. *Dams were built on the Salt & Gila Rivers in Arizona in the 1920s?*
2. *Executive Order 9066 was enacted February 19, 1942?*
3. *Port Chicago experienced a munitions explosion on July 17, 1944?*
4. *The Civil Rights Act of 1964 and Voting Rights Act of 1965 were signed?*
5. *Refugees from the Vietnam War emigrated to the U.S. in the 1970s and 1980s?*
6. *Which of these events were experienced by your patients? What impact do you think it had?*

It is thought that events of the recent past have the most impact on our lives. Why? The answer may lie in the fact that if we were alive during that time our response to the events was personalized. In addition we saw and interpreted each event though our cultural lens. If you were a Native American living in the Southwest, the building of dams impacted your family's ability to farm the land. If you were a Japanese American living on the west coast, loss of business and property due to the enactment of Executive Order 9066 (National Archives) is part of your memory. As an African American, the Civil Rights movement and struggle to obtain equal rights were witnessed in the marches and protests. Each person takes a recent event and internalizes it. Memories may include wariness of government and of those in healthcare institutions. As we reflect on our patient population, we realize that, seen through their eyes, the story may take a different perspective. Let's take a brief look at each.

Construction of dams in the Southwestern portion of the United States had a significant health impact on the Native American nations residing in that area. By 1930 dams had been erected on the Salt and Gila rivers of Arizona. Land once used by the local tribes for farming and fishing was no longer available, and those activities came to an abrupt halt. No longer able to provide for themselves, Native Americans grew to rely on government food subsidies and a sedentary lifestyle.

Japanese Internment followed the bombing of Pearl Harbor December 7, 1941. On February 19, 1942, President Roosevelt signed Executive Order 9066, authorizing the Secretary of War to define military areas "from which any or all persons may be excluded as deemed necessary or desirable." The only significant opposition would come from the Quakers (Society of Friends) and the ACLU (American Civil Liberties Union). More than 122,000 Japanese, many of them citizens of the United States, were forced to live in makeshift housing predominately in the high desert areas away from the Pacific coastline. Manzanar, a site in the Owens Valley, was home to many who had previously lived and owned property and profitable businesses on the west coast. When I toured this site, it became abundantly clear that sanitary and health conditions were questionable. There was little room for privacy. Release from these sites came at the conclusion of World War II. On February 18, 1999, the Justice Department installed a $1.6 billion reparation program for ethnic Japanese interned in American camps during World War II.

12

The Port Chicago Naval Magazine explosion occurred on July 17, 1944. Of the three hundred and twenty killed, two hundred and two were African American. Following the event two hundred and fifty African Americans refused to return to work, citing unsafe conditions. Fifty leaders were identified, charged with mutiny, and imprisoned. In 1946 they were released without amnesty. Finally in 1992, a pardon was granted to Freddie Meeks, one of the last two survivors. In the San Francisco Chronicle (Franko, 2007) a story appeared marking the anniversary of the event. A woman by the name of Diana McDaniel was featured in the article. She stated that she "heard this story as a child." She was advocating that a center be established because "the story cannot be told enough . . ." Recent history is passed down from one generation to the next. It had been sixty years since that event, but the story continued to be told.

The Civil Rights Act of 1964 and the **Voting Rights Act of 1965** were enacted to ensure the rights of all people of the United States. It had been a hundred years since the passage of the 13th, 14th, and 15th amendments, and yet in some parts of the country discriminatory practices were still prevalent. Separate schools and separate entrances for blacks and other minorities had been the norm. Separate hospitals were set up in the late 1880s at the request of the American Medical Association and were in existence until the late 1970s. Separate, however, did not equate with equal services.

The Tuskegee study, which began in 1941, engendered a great deal of distrust of those conducting health research. Participants of this study, African American men, were not provided treatment for syphilis, even though there was a known cure at the time. The hesitancy to seek care may be part of the reason for health disparities found in the African American population today. The study is a prime example that has, for some, led to mistrust of most healthcare professionals.

Manuel Pablo fought with the Americans to protect the Philippines during World War II and participated in the Bataan Death March. At the time he was promised citizenship, a pension and medical benefits, along with resident rights for himself and his children. In a recent article (McAvoy 2007) Mr. Pablo stated that those rights were not realized until 1990 with a revision of the Immigration Act of 1964, which now allows him to bring only one family member to the United States. His other children have been on the wait list for a visa for thirteen years. In her book, *The Spirit Catches You and You Fall Down*, Anne Fadimen (1996) cites the belief of some Hmong men who served with the United States military during the Vietnam War that they, too, would receive veteran benefits following their emigration to America. That did not prove to be a reality. As HCPs, we can help to change a negative experience into a positive one by recognizing their contribution to American society and honoring their individual cultures.

Today ~ being present with the present

History has a way of repeating itself. We, as HCPs, have the opportunity to change the course of events, especially when it comes to the care and treatment of our patient population. Acknowledging the fact that the persons we serve may not trust the health system, we are in a unique position to dialog about this with them. We must recognize that injustices have occurred, and continue to address issues of prejudice and discrimination when we see them. The journey to cultural competence begins with awareness that past events may influence present encounters with patients and colleagues as well. Realizing that these events may have occurred three hundred years ago, sixty years ago, or yesterday, admonishes us to be vigilant in all our encounters, communications, and actions.

Resources

Campinha-Bacote, J. (2008). People of African American heritage. In L.D. Purnell, B.J. Paulanka (Eds.) *Transcultural Health Care: A Culturally Competent Approach*. (3rd Ed.). Philadelphia PA: F. A. Davis.

Center for Disease Control and Prevention. U.S. Public Health Service Syphilis Study at Tuskegee. Retrieved November 24, 2009, from www.cdc.gov/tuskegee

Cherry, B., Giger, J. N. (2008). African Americans. In Giger, J. N., Davidhizar, R. E. (Eds.) *Transcultural Nursing: Assessment and Intervention*. (5th Ed.) St Louis, MO: Mosby/Elsevier

Conti, K. M. (2006). Diabetes prevention in Indian country: Developing nutrition models to tell the story of food-system change. *Journal of Transcultural Nursing*. (17)3, 234-245.

Fadiman, A. (1996). *The Spirit Catches You and You Fall Down*. New York: Farrar, Straus and Giroux.

Falicov, C.J. (2005). Mexican Families. In McGoldrick, M., Giordano, J. Garcia-Preto, N. (Eds) *Ethnicity & Family Therapy*. (3rd Ed.). New York: Guilford Press.

Farmworkers Organization. The Bracero Program. Retrieved August 2, 2009, from www.farmworkers.org/bracero

Franko, K. (2007). New bill keeps Port Chicago's story alive. San Francisco Chronicle. July 30, 2007.

Giger, J. N., Appel, S. J., Davidhizar, R. E., Davis, C. (2008). Church and spirituality in the lives of the African American community. *Journal of Transcultural Nursing*. (19)4, 375-383.

Giordano, J., McGoldrick, M. (2005). European Families: An Overview. In McGoldrick, M., Giordano, J. Garcia-Preto, N. (Eds) *Ethnicity & Family Therapy*. (3rd Ed.). New York: Guilford Press.

Gonzalez, E. W., Owen, D. C., Christina, M., Esperat, R. (2008). Mexican Americans. In Giger, J. N., Davidhizar, R. E. (Eds). *Transcultural Nursing: Assessments and Interventions*. (5th Ed.) St Louis, MO: Mosby/Elsevier

Hanley, C. E. (2008). Navajos. In Giger, J. N., Davidhizar, R. E. (Eds). *Transcultural Nursing: Assessment and Intervention*. (5th Ed.). pp. 276- 299. St Louis, MO: Mosby/Elsevier.

Hines, P. M., Boyd-Franklin, N.. (2005). African American Families. In McGoldrick, M., Giordano, J. Garcia-Preto, N. (Eds) *Ethnicity & Family Therapy*. (3rd Ed.). New York: Guilford Press.

Hodgins, O., Hodgins, D. (2008). Navajo Indians. In Purnell, L. D., Paulanka, B. J. (Eds) *Transcultural Health Care: A Culturally Competent Approach*. (3rd Ed.). pp. 279-283 Philadelphia, PA: F. A. Davis Company.

Lee, E. Mock, M.R.. (2005). Chinese Families. In McGoldrick, M., Giordano, J. Garcia-Preto, N. (Eds) *Ethnicity & Family Therapy*. (3rd Ed.). New York: Guilford Press

Leung, P.K., Boehnlein, J. (2005). Vietnamese Families. In McGoldrick, M., Giordano, J. Garcia-Preto, N. (Eds) *Ethnicity & Family Therapy*. (3rd Ed.). New York: Guilford Press

Malthus, T. (1798). Essay on Principles of Population. Retrieved on July 1, 2009, from www.espy.org/books/malthus/population

Mann, C. (2005). 1491: New Revelations about Americans before Columbus. New York: Random House.

McAvoy, A. (2007). Aging Filipino WWII Veterans forced to live apart from famiies. *San Francisco Chronicle*. March 18, 2007.

McGill, D.W., Pearce, J.K.. (2005). AmericanFamilies with English Ancestors from the Colonial Era: Anglo American. In McGoldrick, M., Giordano, J. Garcia-Preto, N. (Eds) *Ethnicity & Family Therapy*. (3rd Ed.). New York: Guilford Press.

McGoldrick, M, Giordano, J., Garcia-Preto, N. (2005). *Ethnicity & Family Therapy*. (3rd Ed.). New York: Guilford Press

National Archives. U.S. Constitution. Retrieved March 20, 2010, National Archives Executive Order 9066. Retrieved August 2, 2009 from www.archieves.com

National Park Service. Ellis Island. Retrieved October 3, 2009, from www.nps.gov

Nowak, T. T. (2003). People of Vietnamese heritage. In Purnell, L. D., Paulanka, B. J. (Eds.) *Transcultural Health Care: A Culturally Competent Approach*. (2nd Ed.). Philadelphia PA: F. A. Davis.

Purnell, L. (2008). People of Vietnamese heritage. In Purnell, L. D., Paulanka, B. J. (Eds.) *Transcultural Health Care: A Culturally Competent Apporach*. (3rd Ed.). Philadelphia PA: F. A. Davis.

Spector, R. (2009). *Cultural Diversity in Health and Illness*. (7th Ed.). New Jersey: Pearson,Prentice Hall.

Staisak, D. (1991). Culture care theory with Mexican Americans in an urban context. In Leininger, M. M. (Ed.). *Culture care diversity & universality: A theory in nursing*. New York: National League for Nursing Press.

Stauffer, R. Y. (2008). Vietnamese Americans. In Giger, J. N., Davidhizar, R.E. (Eds.) *Transcultural Nursing: Assessment and Intervention*. (5th Ed.) St Louis, MO: Mosby/Elsevier

Penner, L. A., Dovidio, J. F., Edmondson, D., Dailey, R. K., Markova, T., Albrecht, T. L., Gaertner, S. L. (2009). The experience of discrimination and Black-White health disparities in medical care. *Journal of Black Psychology.* (35)2, 181-203.

Public Broadcasting System. (2008). Unnatural Causes: Is inequality making us sick?

Public Broadcasting System. (2009). Our National Parks. United States Department of State. Public Diplomacy & Public Affairs. Retrieved on November 24, 2009, from www.state.gov

United States Department of the Interior. Bureau of Indian Affairs. November 24, 2009, from www.cr.nps.gov

United States Department of the Interior. Ellis Island: History and Culture. Retrieved October 20, 2009, from www.nps.gov/ellis/historyculture

Wang, Y., Purnell, L. (2008) People of Chinese Heritage. In Purnell, L. D., Paulanka, B. J. (Eds). *Transcultural health care: A Culturally Competent Approach.* (3rd Ed.), Philadelphia: F. A. Davis.

Warne, D. (2006). Research and educational approaches to reducing health disparities among American Indians and Alaskan natives. *Journal ofTranscultural Nursing.* (17)3, 266-271.

Xu, Y, Chang, K. (2008). Chinese Americans. In Giger, J. N., Davidhizar, R. E. (Eds). *Transcultural Nursing: Assessments and Interventions.* (5th Ed.), St Louis, MO: Mosby/Elsevier.

Zoucha, R., Zamarripa, C. (2008). People of Mexican Heritage. In Purnell, L. D., Paulanka, B. J. (Eds). *Transcultural Health Care: A Culturally Competent Approach.* (3rd Ed.) Philadelphia: F. A. Davis.

Growing More Diverse . . . Trends Over Time | 3

"...demographics are only as good as the people who fill out the forms"
– A seminar participant

This was the response I received during a recent seminar. A participant, sitting at the back of the room and acting as though he wished he were somewhere else, startled me with his response. But, he was right! The census data is only as reliable as the people who fill out the forms. Much has been written about the hesitancy of some to provide the information because of illiteracy, distrust, or apathy toward the process. What the census does reflect is trends over time.

The census was written into the United States Constitution of 1789 and stated:

Article I, Section 2
of the Constitution of the United States
"Representation and direct Taxes shall be apportioned among the several States which may be included within this Union, according to their respective Numbers . . . The actual Enumeration shall be made within three Years after the first Meeting of the Congress of the United States, and within every subsequent Term of ten Years, in such Manner as they shall by Law direct."

It came about because the Revolutionary War created a debt. No longer receiving support from England, the Congress looked to the new states to share the debt and to provide revenue. In addition, it gave an accurate picture of the current population, which also determined representation in Congress. The initial census included "white" males and excluded Indians who were not taxed. Slaves were each counted as 3/5 of a person. Each succeeding census in the 1800s saw a 25% to 30% growth in the population of the United States. The 3/5 slave designation was repealed in 1865 with the passage of the 14th Amendment. In 1913 the 16th Amendment authorized directed taxation of the individual which ended the census' role in determining state taxation.

The current census includes White and Black (African American, Negro); those identifying themselves as American Indian or Alaskan Native can list their tribe affiliation; Spanish/Hispanic/Latino can list Mexican, Mexican American, Chicano, Puerto Rican, Cuban or write in another group. Those of Asian or Southeast Asian heritage are also given an opportunity to write in another race. So, yes, we definitely see trends over time, and that enables us to reflect on the changes within our community and country.

U.S. Census Bureau Population 2008 Estimate

Black ~ African American	12.8%
American Indian/Alaskan Native	1.0%
Asian	4.5%
Native Hawaiian/ Pacific Islander	0.2%
Hispanic ~ Latino	15.4%
White ~ Non Hispanic	65.6%

Who fits in what category . . . interesting!

According to the U.S. Census Bureau (2000) the "concept of race reflects self-identification by people according to the race or races with which they most closely identify. These categories are sociopolitical constructs and should not be interpreted as being scientific or anthropological in nature. Furthermore, the race categories include both racial and national-origin groups."

The following race classifications are used by the U.S. Census Bureau and are consistent with the *"Revisions to the Standards for the Classification of Federal Data on Race and Ethnicity"* issued in 1997 by the Office of Management and Budget. Each group is listed below and includes both race and national-origin as the defining factors.

White: a person having origins in any of the original peoples of Europe, the Middle East or North Africa. It includes people who indicate their race as "White" or other, such as Irish, German, Lebanese, Arab, and Polish.

Black or African American: a person having origins in any of the Black racial groups of Africa. It includes those who indicate their race as "Black, African American, or Negro" or provide written entries such as Nigerian, Afro American, Kenyan, and Haitian.

American Indian and Alaskan Native: a person having origins in any of the original peoples of North and South America (including Central America) and who maintain tribal affiliation or community attachment.

Asian: a person having origins in any of the original peoples of the Far East, Southeast Asia, or the Indian subcontinent including for example, Cambodia, China, India, Japan, Korea, Malaysia, Pakistan, the Philippine Islands, Thailand and Vietnam. It includes Asian Indian, Chinese, Filipino, Korean, Japanese, Vietnamese, and Other Asian.

Native Hawaiian and Other Pacific Islander: a person having origins in any of the original peoples of Hawaii, Guam, Samoa, or other Pacific Islands. It includes people who indicate their race as Native Hawaiian, Guamanian or Chamorro, Samoan, and Other Pacific Islander.

Reflective exercise: Who lives here . . . works here . . .?
1. *What is the demographic make-up of your community?*
2. *Is this a change from ten or twenty years ago?*
3. *Do you have an immigrant or refugee population?*
4. *Are healthcare professionals representative of your patient population?*

Immigrants and Health

The article, *America's Diversity at the Beginning of the 21st Century: Reflections from Census 2000,* written by Audrey Singer (2002) of the Brooking Institution, explores the similarities and differences between the immigrants arriving at the beginning of the 20th century and those coming at the end. In the early 1900s Southern and Eastern Europeans constituted the majority of immigrants, 14.5 million, admitted to the United States. The end of the century found that the majority of groups came from Asia, Latin America, the Caribbean, and Africa. Singer states that "both periods – the beginning and the end of the century – have been characterized by a

21

broad restructuring of the nation's economy, from agricultural to industry in the early period and in the later period from manufacturing to services and information technology."

More than a million immigrants come to this country annually, many seeking a better life for themselves and their families. There are more than 12 million undocumented immigrants in the United States. While this constitutes less than 0.4% of the total population it seems to generate the majority of attention with regard to healthcare and employment.

Let's look at the health of one immigrant group. The Public Broadcasing System documentary (PBS) *Unnatural Causes . . . Is Inequality Making Us Sick* (2008), cites that Latino immigrants have the *best health* in the country – better health than the wealthiest. The authors hypothesized two reasons for this finding: (1) only the healthiest make it across the border; and (2) the role of strong cohesive ties with family and strong social networks that form a protective barrier. Unfortunately, though, within one generation those health advantages decline. Acculturation, adapting to the American way of life, may lead to intergenerational stress and a loss of connection with family. The health protective benefits begin to wane and health issues such as obesity, diabetes, and heart disease rise.

<u>Reflective exercise</u>: **Immigrants in your community**
1. *Who are the immigrants in your community?*
2. *What ways does it challenge you to care for this population?*
3. *What resources are available . . . for you . . . for your patients?*
4. *Has your organization provided you with continuing education programs about caring for diverse populations?*

HCP Demographics . . . are they changing?

As the demographic landscape continues to change the challenge facing HCPs is providing culturally sensitive and competent care. The current HCP population, however, is predominantly white. The following data highlights the numbers: Health Resources and Services Administration (HRSA 2000) highlights the registered nurse population, the Office of Minority Health (2004), the physician population; and the Center for Workforce Studies & NASW Center for Workforce Studies (2004), the social worker demographics. The numbers are rounded up.

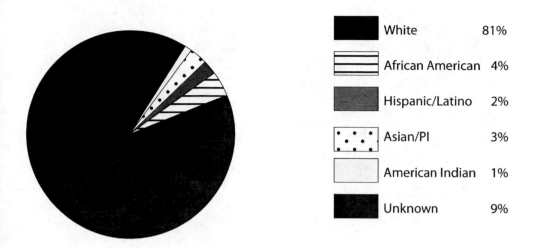

■	White	81%
≡	African American	4%
▨	Hispanic/Latino	2%
⠐⠂	Asian/PI	3%
□	American Indian	1%
■	Unknown	9%

Figure 3-1: Registered Nurse Demographics

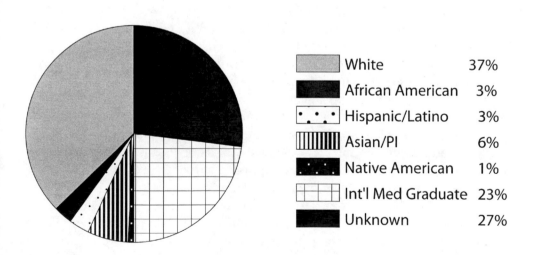

▨	White	37%
■	African American	3%
⠐⠂	Hispanic/Latino	3%
▥	Asian/PI	6%
▨	Native American	1%
▦	Int'l Med Graduate	23%
■	Unknown	27%

Figure 3-2: 2004 Physician Demographics

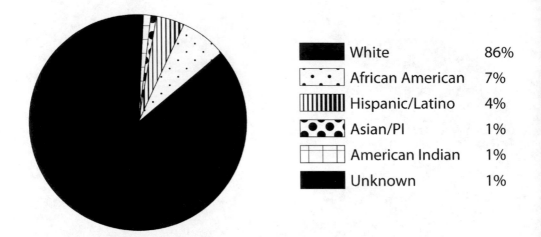

■	White	86%
⬚	African American	7%
▥	Hispanic/Latino	4%
⬤	Asian/PI	1%
▦	American Indian	1%
■	Unknown	1%

Figure 3-3: 2004 Social Workers Demographics

Finding the future HCP . . .

According to the National League of Nursing (2008), 24% of all nursing graduates nationally are minorities: Black 10.3%, Hispanic 7%, Asian/PI 4.5%, American Indian 1%, and other 3.7%. Enrollment in medical schools, similar to that of registered nurses, shows minimal increase for all minority groups with the exception of Hispanics, which is declining. Unfortunately, this leads to an under representation of bilingual and bicultural HCPs in hospitals, clinics and home health programs.

Legislation titled *Closing the Health Care Gap*, passed by Congress in 2004, addressed the need for more diversity in the healthcare field by funding outreach programs to attract minority students. Yet, why does there continue to be a disparity in the HCP demographics? For those minority students in high school considering a career in healthcare, the educational level and income of their parents may be a factor. Navigating the college application process and facing limited funding can adversely affect their ability to follow their dream. Language proficiency for students who have been here less than five years may seem like an insurmountable obstacle.

In the article *Racial/Ethnic Disparities in Nursing* (2001), Coffman, Rosenoff, and Grumback hypothesize that one reason for low enrollment of minority groups in college may be due to low rates of high school graduation.

According to the Brooking Institute Civil Rights Report of 2004, there is a fifty percent dropout rate for African Americans, Latinos, and American Indians. Those who do pursue higher education may be less likely than whites to obtain a degree in nursing. If this is the current reality, then what can we do as HCPs to change that trend? It may be as simple as serving as a role model to the young people we meet or helping present at health fairs in their schools. Share your passion for what you do and let students know they can make a difference in the lives of others. Getting young people interested and excited earlier, rather than later, may be the key to increasing the diversity of HCPs in the future. When we inspire and motivate, young people listen and are encouraged to further their education.

Other barriers for future the HCP . . . perhaps

Cultural beliefs and values may influence one's decision to enter the healthcare field. Those in the American Indian culture may view nursing as undesirable because it involves being around sick people. Olivia Still and David Hodgins (2003) share that most of the nurses in the Indian Health Service are not American Indian. They went on to note that "it is frequently said that if an American Indian became a physician, he must not be 'traditional'. . . therefore many Navajo are suspicious of American Indian physicians" (p. 292).

Those who value harmony and are more collectivistic than individualistic, such as the native Hawaiian, may view the classroom and clinical areas as competitive, aggressive, and unwelcoming. At a recent Transcultural Nursing conference, a registered nurse, who was also native Hawaiian, shared the story of her university experience. In the classroom she said, "None of the Hawaiians would ever speak, but when they attended separate classes just for their group they never stopped talking and sharing." She felt intimidated by the individual competition and was more comfortable working as a group. This style is consistent with her cultural values and educational practices. That experience was ten years ago, but she shared it with me as if it happened yesterday.

Another limitation may be related religious values and beliefs that prevent care to a person of the opposite sex (Muslim and Orthodox Jew), or working certain days of the week, such as the Sabbath (Seventh Day Adventist, Muslim, Orthodox Jew). These limitations may restrict the ability of the student to become a full participant in the educational process.

25

Creating a welcoming environment

Acknowledging the need and the opportunity for a more diverse healthcare staff, we need to recognize the ambiance of the academic arena that sets the stage for student success. Clinical experience challenges the students to transition academic knowledge to the clinical practice. Do you remember your first day as a student or as a new graduate? Even though we were apprehensive, our expectations were high. The encouragement we received from the veteran staff helped to make it a success. The most important thing we can do is to provide a supportive and welcoming environment.

Moving on . . .

As a country we are becoming more diverse. We are a destination for many immigrants and refugees. This will continue. Healthcare professionals, at this time, do not reflect the current population. As healthcare professionals, we grapple with the unknown, the uncertainty, and the challenges of working and caring for people from diverse ethnic, cultural, and religious backgrounds. My colleagues say "it's about the patient . . . the patient comes first." We need do what is necessary to provide care and restore health and wellbeing. Are we ready?

Resources

Association of American Medical Colleges. (2006). American Needs a
    More Diverse Physician Workforce. AAMC: Washington D.C.
Coffman, J. M., Rosenoff, E., Grumbach. K. (2001). Racial/Ethnic
    Disparities in Nursing. *Health Affairs.* May/June 263-264.
Hendricks, T. (2009). Kids Boost Diversity as State Ages. *San Francisco
    Chronicle.*
Lipson, J., Dibble, S., (2005). Culture & Clinical Care. San Francisco, CA:
    UCSF Nursing Press
National League of Nursing. (2008). Number of nursing school graduates.
    Retreived from www.nln.org
NASW Center for Workforce Studies. (2006). Licensed Social Workers in
    the United States, 2004.
Olvera, M. L. (2005). Fact Sheet: Census Schedules and Ethnic
    Classification Chicago IL: Cultural Marketing Communication and
    Urban Reach Public Relations.
    www.culturalmarketingcommunications.com
Public Broadcasting System. (2008). Unnatural causes . . . Is inequality
    making us sick?
Purnell, L. D., Paulanka, B. J. (2008). *Transcultural Health Care: A
    Culturally Competent Approach.* (3rd Ed.). Philadelphia, PA: F. A.
    Davis Company
Singer, A. (2002). America's Diversity at the Beginning of the 21st
    Century: Reflections from Census 2000. Brooking Institute:
    Washington D.C. 1-15.
Still, O, Hodgins, D. (2003). Navajo Indians. In Purnell, L., Paulanka, B.J. (Eds)
    Transcultural Health Care: A Culturally Ccompetent Aapproach. (2rd Ed).
    Philadelphia, PA: F.A. Davis Company
Spector, R. (2009). *Cultural Diversity in Health and Illness.* (7th Ed.). New
    Jersey: Pearson,Prentice Hall.
U.S. Census Bureau. (2003). Language Use and English-Speaking Ability:
    2000. U.S. Department of Commerce. Economics and Statistic
    Administration.
U.S. Census Bureau. (2005). Facts for Features: National Nurses Week and
    National Hospital Week. Washington D.C.
U.S. Department of Health and Human Services. (2005). Minorities in
    Medicine: An Ethnic and Cultural Challenge for Physician Training.
    Council on Graduate Medical Education 17th Report. 1-62.

U.S. Department of Health Resources and Services Administration. (2004). The Registered Nurse Population: National Sample Survey of Registered Nurses. Retrieved May 2, 2009, from http:www.hrsa.gov/healthworkforce/rnsurvey

It's Time to Talk About Race, Prejudice and Discrimination | 4

*"But race is an issue that I believe this nation
cannot afford to ignore right now . . . "*
— *Barack Obama ~ March 3, 2008*

Most people find racism, prejudice, and discrimination difficult topics at best and would rather avoid them or pretend that they don't exist: but they do exist. Each one may influence a person's access to care, treatment, and health outcomes. A recent documentary titled *Unnatural Causes: Is Inequality Making Us Sick?* aired by PBS in 2009 believed that constant exposure to racism and discrimination increases stress and has a negative impact on one's health. The physiological response is for the body to release large amounts of cortisol from the adrenals. While this is helpful in a "fight or flight" situation, continuous release of this hormone results in an elevation of the blood pressure and blood sugar while lowering the immune system. So, yes, we need to talk about this subject, to identify biases and to eliminate prejudice, discrimination, and racism for many reasons, including our own health.

Race . . . when did it begin?

Let's look at the word race from a historical perspective. The term was constructed in the mid to late 1800s during a time when all things were being categorized, thus systematically explaining their surroundings. Race is a social construct, not necessarily based on ethnicity, but more significantly on the color of one's skin (2006 American Anthropological Association). Scientists used the taxonomic system to classify humans during this period of time, positing that there were biological differences in capabilities and intellect. It provided the legitimacy for laws that promoted social inequalities, thus disenfranchising groups of people such as African Americans, Native Americans, immigrants and others.

Racism and other uncomfortable subjects

Racism, unfortunately alive and well, is demonstrated through acts of prejudice and discrimination. It may be subtle. It may be overt. Think about a time when you experienced some form of racism. How did you feel? What did you do? How did it change your perspective of the individual or organization involved? Dr. Adewale Troutman, Public Health and Wellness Director in Louisville, Kentucky, shares his story in the 2009 PSB series *Unnatural Causes . . . Is Inequality Making Us Sick?* He serves a county populated by Kentucky's poor and disenfranchised. Yet, as an African American he has experienced racism where he lives and works. "There are times when I get on the elevator and the elderly white woman clutches her purse . . . or every time I walk down the aisles of a certain store someone follows me to make sure I am not stealing anything. What they don't know about me is that I live in an affluent part of the city and hold two degrees," he said in the documentary previously cited. Many people face this every day, and as HCP our antennas must be attuned to be aware of incidents that occur in our workplace.

Let's review the following definitions and reflect on their impact on ourselves, our patients, and our colleagues.
- Race ~ a sociopolitical construct; refers to the genetic, biological differences such as skin color, or other outward physical appearances
- Racism ~ a belief that all members of each race possess certain characteristics or abilities specific to that race; especially to distinguish it as inferior or superior to another race or races
- Ethnicity ~ a group that shares a common history, culture, values and beliefs, linguistic or religious beliefs along with other characteristics that form a shared identity
- Prejudice ~ a set of rigid and unfavorable attitudes toward a particular individual or group that is formed without consideration of facts
- Discrimination ~ a set of attitudes that often leads to discrimination, the differential treatment of individuals or groups based on categories such as race, ethnicity, gender, sexual orientation, social class, religious affiliation, immigrant status

- Cultural bias ~ believing that one's personal beliefs and values are superior
- Cultural imposition ~ imposing one's cultural beliefs and values on another in an intrusive manner
- Ethnocentrism ~ the belief, assumption or perception that oneself or group is superior to another; an inherent superiority

Forming opinions . . . it begins early in life

We learn biases at an early age. Prior to the ability to differentiate between races of people, observation and socialization with our family of origin lay the groundwork for establishing biases. Before the age of five a child learns attitudes and beliefs about the differences between people and the things in their environment. Recently, a five-year-old child whose mother is white and father is black shared an "aha" moment when he said to his mother, "I know who I am . . . it's kinda like ice cream. I am chocolate, because I am dark; you are vanilla because you are white; and Sammy (his younger brother) is," and here he paused, "Sammy is marble fudge, because he is more white than black." He had selected something that he loved, ice cream, and used that model to provide positive attributes to his mother and brother. By the age of ten this same child will likely form attitudes and beliefs, positive and negative. This is what his world tells him about the "other" and he begins to believe it to be true. It is not until adulthood, however, that one has the opportunity to change previous biases, behaviors, and stereotypical opinions about others.

Bias . . . Naming it . . . Saying it . . . Dissolving it . . .

Bias, negative or positive, conscious or unconscious, is a belief about a particular group of people. This then translates into stereotyping, a firmly held belief that influences how one interacts with another.

Reflective exercise: List your first positive and negative thoughts after reading each one:
1. *African American - college - male - dreadlocks*
2. *Asian - math - herbs - driving*
3. *White - pregnant - poverty - alone*
4. *Native American - overweight - casino - pride*
5. *Woman - executive - African American - new*
6. *Elderly - new hire - thrifty - organized*

What was the first thought that came into your head after reading each one? Did some of these responses surprise you? If this had been done using a group setting, different perspectives would have been presented. Those responses can help us to widen our views and open us to a new way of thinking, thus hopefully eliminating previously held biases and stereotypes.

Stereotyping as defined by Webster's 1950 Merriam Dictionary refers to the use of a mold to make a plate . . . lacking originality or individuality . . . to repeat without variation; to hackney. The 2009 version defines stereotyping as "oversimplification of the typical characteristics of a person or thing." The difference of sixty years takes the term to a new level. Research in social psychology indicates that stereotyping is a *universal cognitive function* (IOM 2002). It is not unique to one group of people, one religious sect, or one socioeconomic group. It is universal and worldwide. On a recent trip to Costa Rica for a Spanish immersion program, mi madre told me about the *Nicas* and the *Ticas*. Still not well versed in Spanish, I asked for clarification. She informed me, en Español, that the *Ticas* were Costa Ricans and the *Nicas* were Nicaraguans. The *Nicas* were coming across the border to use Costa Rica's health facilities, schools, and welfare system. Being naïve, I asked "How can you tell the difference?" She adamantly shared, "They all (she placed great emphasis on the word all) look and talk the same." A recent documentary on immigrants entering Botswana from Zimbabwe depicted a similar view that these immigrants were taking jobs and using resources. How could they tell the difference between those from Botswana and those from Zimbabwe? The response from one woman: "They smell different." In her worldview it was fact. What we see and what we know may be very different.

Why do we do this? Initially, it may provide confidence in our ability to control the situation or possibly be used to respond when facts are not readily available. Unfortunately, it may create and promote validation of opinions that are prejudiced. The Institute of Medicine report, *Unequal Treatment* (2002), states that research in cognitive reasoning and psychology reveals that stereotypes:

- Are automatically activated ~ generated without conscious effort
- Are held by people who truly believe they do not judge others
- Affect how we process and recall information about others
- Guide our expectations and perceptions and shape our personal interaction.

Proverbial "Iceberg"

The proverbial "iceberg" is a frequently used image that helps us to understand that much of what we do not know about patients and colleagues is beneath the water line, yet to be discovered. Initial encounters may evoke positive and negative opinions. Our patients may have an iceberg perspective of us as well. Are biases at work or stereotypes forming? Based on previous encounters with other health professionals, the patient may draw on her memory as well to form an opinion. It is vital that we as HCPs understand that our patients present to us with their biases as well.

The more knowledge HCPs have about cultural values, beliefs, and healthcare practices of various ethnic groups, the more likely they are to have established respectful and trusting relationships with patients and colleagues.

- Knowledge replaces stereotyping.
- Positive and respectful encounters replace stereotyping.
- Welcoming environments replace stereotyping.

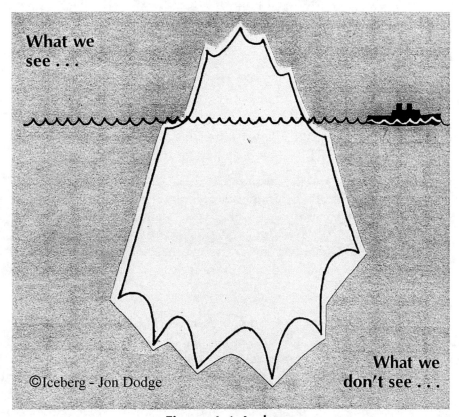

Figure 4-1: Iceberg

Overcoming bias in the every day

Biases can lead to making decisions that negatively affect future encounters. So what are the steps one should take to elevate consciousness, address the bias, and then eliminate it? *Reducing Unconscious Bias* (2009), an article by Sondra Thiederman, Ph.D. (copyright 2009 Sondra Thiederman/Cross-Cultural Communications; www.thiederman.com, used with permission), offers the following suggestions:

Step 1: Become aware of your bias
- Identify that first thought that comes to mind
- when encountering someone different from yourself
- What assumptions are you making?
- Example:

Step 2: Examine your thoughts
- Look at your reaction and think ~ "would I feel the same way about the meaning of this incident if that person were from a different group?"
- Is this related to a previous experience with the group involved?
- Is your assumption is incorrect
- Example:

Step 3: Dissect your bias to reveal its weak foundation
- Was the original source of my bias reliable?
- Was it a self-fulfilling prophecy or the filter of expectation?

Step 4: Fake it until you make it
- Make a list of the things your bias about how people communicate is causing you to do and the consequences of these behaviors
- Substitute behavior and visualize positive consequences
- The more positive one views another, the better response from that individual and the more positive the experience for all concerned

Thiederman suggests *Bias Spotter Partnerships* which is based on the following four principles: (1) awareness of our biases is the best first step toward resolution, (2) human beings resist identifying our own biases because we feel that having a bias means we are bad people, (3) the stress and rush of the workplace deprives us of the luxury of spotting the tiny clues to bias that our behavior and thoughts reveal, and (4) team members can serve as trusted aids in bringing about awareness of our biases. This approach can be used in the workplace and thus translated into a collaborative effort in which all members of the team/staff identify biases in the spirit of mutual support without being accusatory. Confidentiality is important as well. For the next couple of weeks, notice the first thought that comes into your mind when encountering someone different from yourself or that patient with a long history of negative encounters with HCP. Use the four steps outlined to identify, examine, dissect and substitute previous behavior and thoughts. You will see new and positive outcomes. Attitude follows behavior.

Ethnocentrism & Cultural Acceptance

Juxtaposing these two terms may seem an oxymoron, but in reality one may actually lead to another. Ethnocentrism, according to W. G. Summer in the early part of the 20th century, was defined as "the view of things in which one's own group is the center of everything and all others are scaled and rated from it." (Capell, Dean, Veenstra 2008, p. 121) It is interesting to note that he suggests that persons then hold onto their beliefs, values, and folkways in order to protect themselves from foreigners. It was a survival strategy to maintain their identities.

Cultural values and practices that we learn as children through observation, communication, and socialization can lead to ethnocentric beliefs. Becoming aware that one has beliefs of superiority over another individual or group provides the first step in the journey to ethnorelativism, a belief that another's cultural beliefs, values, and ways of living in the world are on an equal par with one's own. This transition does not happen in a day, a week, or a year. It does not happen because of one incident, one encounter, or one "aha" moment. Opportunities to learn about others garners cultural knowledge and moves us from the unconscious ethnocentric thoughts to a conscious decision to make changes that will lead to culturally sensitive and competent healthcare.

Our patients also may hold ethnocentric beliefs about us as well. Expectations may lead to misunderstandings, tension, and uncertainty. It is during these moments that we realize that this is an opportunity to dispel previously held biases and eliminate stereotyping of each other. When we persevere in difficult times, we learn something new about our patients and ourselves.

Now to assessment . . .

Where are you on the river of prejudice and discrimination? This activity allows recognition that your response may vary according to the situation. Visualize yourself in a canoe on a river. Yes, you have a lifejacket on ~ a great metaphor for dealing in uncertainty. There are five potential answers, beginning with promoting racism and discrimination, to level five in which you are a constant voice speaking out against injustice. Where are you?

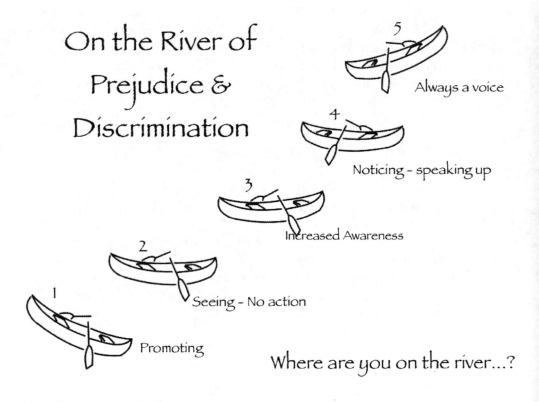

Figure 4-2: On the River

Reflective exercise: **On the scale of 1 - 5 . . . where are you on the river . . . ?**

	1	2	3	4	5
1. *In the clinical setting:*	*1*	*2*	*3*	*4*	*5*
2. *In the staff meeting:*	*1*	*2*	*3*	*4*	*5*
3. *At the supermarket:*	*1*	*2*	*3*	*4*	*5*
4. *At a family gathering:*	*1*	*2*	*3*	*4*	*5*

Where to from here . . .

The process is ongoing. Take the opportunity to attend cultural awareness education seminars that address issues of prejudice, discrimination, and racism in addition to cultural beliefs, values, and practices of various groups. Reviewing policies and procedures, orientation programs, staff evaluations, annual goals and objectives, and the mission statement of the organization can and should be part of this process. It's time to talk about all things uncomfortable!

Resources

American Anthropological Association. (2006). The Story of Race. Retrieved October 5, 2009, from http://www.understandingrace.com

Andrews, M. M., Boyle, J. S. (2008). *Transcultural concepts in nursing care*. (5th Ed.).New York: Lippincott Williams & Wilkins.

Beckles, G. (2008). The intellectual origins of race. Retrieved November 5 2008, from www.suite101.com

Campinha-Bacote, J. (2003). The process of cultural competence in the delivery of healthcare services: A culturally competent model of care. Cincinnati, OH: Transcultural C.A.R.E. Associates.

Capell, J., Dean, E., Veenstra, G. (2008). The relationship between cultural competence and ethnocentrism of healthcare professionals. *Journal of Transcultural Nursing*. (19)2; 121-125.

Galanti, G. (2000). An introduction to cultural differences. *Western Journal of Medicine*. 172:335-336.

Giger, J. N., Davidhizar, R. E. (2008). *Transcultural nursing: Assessment and intervention*. (5th Ed.). St Louis, MO: Mosby/Elsevier

Giger, J., Davidhizar, R., Purnell, L., Harden, J., Phillips, J., Stickland. (2007). American Academy of Nursing Expert Panel Report: Developing cultural competence to eliminate health disparities in ethnic minorities and other vulnerable populations. *Journal of Transcultural Nursing*. (18) 2, 95-102.

Hassouneh-Phillips, D., Beckett, P. (2003). An education in Racism. *Journal of Nursing Education*. (42)6; 258-266.

Leininger, M. M. (1991). *Culture care diversity and universality: A theory of nursing*. New York: National League for Nursing Press.

Leininger, M. M., McFarland, M. R. (2002). *Transcultural nursing: Concepts, theories, research and practice*. (3rd Ed.). New York: McGraw-Hill.

Lipson, J., Dibble, S., (2005). *Culture & Clinical Care* (8th Ed.) San Francisco, CA: UCSF NursingPress:

Mansour, M. (1994). Cultural circles: Application of Family Systems Theory in staff development. *Journal of Nursing Staff Development*. (10)1; 22-26.

McGoldrick, M, Giordano, J., Garcia-Preto, N. (2005). *Ethnicity & Family Therapy*. (3rd Ed.). New York: Guilford Press

Obama, B. (2008). A More Perfect Union. Retrieved on September 14, 2009 from www.huffingtonpost.com

Purnell, L. D., Paulanka, B. J. (2008). *Transcultural health care: A culturally competent approach.* (3rd Ed.). Philadelphia, PA: F. A. Davis Company.

Smedley, B., Stith, A., Nelson, A. (2002). Unequal treatment: Confronting racial and ethnic disparities in healthcare. Institute of Medicine. Washington D.C.: The National Academies Press.

Spector, R. (2009). *Cultural Diversity in Health and Illness.* (7th Ed.). New Jersey: Pearson,Prentice Hall.

Spence, D. (2001). Prejudice, paradox, and possibility: Nursing people from cultures other than one's own. *Journal of Transcultural Nursing.* (12) 2, 100-106.

Sutherland, L. (2002). Ethnocentrism in a pluristic society: a concept anaylsis. *Journal of Transcultural Nursing.* (13)4; 274-281.

Thiederman, S. (2009). Reducing Unconscious Bias. Retrieved October 2009 from www.thiederman.com

Thiederman, S. (2009). Aren't you overreacting just a bit? Retrieved August 2009 from www.thiederman.com

Thiederman, S. (2009). Leading Biased Free: Capturing Your Career Advantage. Retrieved October 2008 from www.thiederman.com

Healthcare Disparities . . . What Is Making Us Sick?

5

These statistics, drawn from the National Healthcare Disparities report of 2003, were used by former Senators William Frist of Tennessee and Senator Mary Landrieu of Louisiana to highlight the need for healthcare reform.

General
- American Indians/Alaska Natives, African Americans, and Hispanics are more likely to report poor health.
- On average, African Americans and American Indians/Alaska Natives have higher overall rates of death than any other racial or ethnic group.

Breast and Cervical Cancer
- Although deaths caused by breast cancer have decreased among white women since 1980s, in 2001 African American women had a 34% higher rate of death from breast cancer than white women.
- In addition, women of racial and ethnic minorities are less likely to receive a Pap test, and thus have higher rates of cervical cancer.

Cardiovascular Disease
- African Americans have the highest rate of high blood pressure of all groups and tend to develop it younger than other groups.
- Counties in rural Appalachia have the second highest death rate in the nation from heart disease. Nearly 44% of these residents have never had a serum cholesterol check.

Diabetes
- Among adults aged 20 or older, African Americans are twice as likely as whites to have diabetes, and American Indians and Alaskan Natives are 2.6 times more likely to have diabetes. Hispanics are 1.9 times more likely to have diabetes.
- African Americans and American Indians have higher rates of diabetes-related complications such as kidney disease and amputations.

HIV/AIDS
- HIV infection is the fifth leading cause of death for people who are 25-34 years old in the United States and is the leading cause of death for African American men in the same age group.
- Although African American and Hispanic persons represent about one-quarter of the country's population, more than half of new AIDS cases reported to the CDC are among these populations.
- Among children, the disparities are even more dramatic, with African American and Hispanic children representing more that 80% of pediatric AIDS cases in 2000.

Infant Mortality
- Infant mortality rates, which are one of the most sensitive indicators of health and well-being, are significantly higher in African American and American Indian/Alaska Native populations.
- Infant mortality among African Americans in 2000 occurred at a rate of 14.1 deaths per 1,000 live births, more than twice the national average.
- The leading causes of infant death include congenital abnormalities, pre-term low birth weight, Sudden Infant Death Syndrome (SIDS), problems related to complications of pregnancy, and respiratory distress syndrome. SIDS deaths among American Indians and Alaskan Natives are 2.3 times the rate for non-Hispanic white infants.

Obesity
- African Americans (66%) and Hispanic adults (62%) are twice as likely to be overweight as Asian/Pacific Islanders (32%). Slightly more than half of white non-Hispanic adults are considered overweight.
- Counties in rural Appalachia have the ninth highest rate of obesity.

- Among African Americans, the proportion of women who are obese is 80% higher than the proportion of men who are obese. This gender difference is also seen among HIspanic women and men, but the percentage of white, non-Hispanic women and men who are obese is about the same.

Vaccines

- In 2001, Hispanics and African Americans aged 65 or older were less likely to receive either influenza or pneumococcal vaccinations.

Reflective exercise: Disparities in health
1. *Did these statistics surprise you?*
2. *Who are the people in your patient/client population?*
3. *Do they reflect the statistics?*
4. *What questions do you need to ask during an assessment?*

These statistics came from the offices of former Senators William Frist of Tennessee and Senator Mary Landrieu of Louisiana. Along with Ted Kennedy, the late Senator from Massachusetts, Frist collaborated on a bill titled, *Closing the Health Care Gap 2004*, which built on a bill of the same title passed in 2000. It acknowledged that in order to eliminate health disparities, changes in the healthcare system must be part of the process. Listed below are five elements needed to close the gap.

1. Improved healthcare quality and data efforts
2. Expanded access to quality healthcare
3. Strong national leadership, cooperation and coordination
4. Professional education, awareness and training
5. Enhanced research

The term "disparity" is defined in the *Oxford Dictionary* as a "great difference." These two words speak clearly about healthcare outcomes. The American Academy of Nursing's Expert Panel defined it as "differences in the incidence, prevalence, mortality, and burden of diseases and other adverse health conditions that exist among specific populations groups in the United States" (Giger et al. 2007, p. 95). When did these disparities begin, and why do they continue, given the vast increase in medical knowledge and technology? Now that we know the facts, how do we increase awareness and change?

The first step is to acknowledge that disparities do exist. Second, we need to identify health conditions in our patient population that are consistent with the statistics. Lastly, we need to promote collaboration between the HCP and the patient to include cultural values, beliefs, and healthcare practices. Change can occur when desire and knowledge are the foundation.

So when did these disparities begin?

Looking back one hundred years or so, it becomes very clear that issues of socioeconomics, racism, and discrimination have played a role in creating health disparities. In the late 1860s, the American Medical Association (AMA) prohibited the use of homeopathic therapies in favor of allopathic therapy. Allopathic therapies embrace "proven" methods that are scientifically based. Around this same time, the AMA prevented women from joining medical societies and practiced segregation. (Spector 2009, p. 95). In addition, Jewish hospitals were built to provide Jewish American interns a place to secure a residency position.

Another landmark event, one that affected the Native American population significantly, was the construction of dams in the Southwest and Midwest. The land where Native Americans had prospered for many centuries was now under water. They were forced to move from their homeland to an area that was incongruous with their lifestyle of hunting, fishing, and farming. Relocation changed everything. To compensate for the loss, government food subsides were started in 1940. The combination of food subsides (lard, flour, peanut butter, cheese) and a now sedentary lifestyle laid the groundwork for health issues, especially diabetes. Trust was affected. Past events, such as broken treaties and loss of land, may have led to a distrust of the government and healthcare systems.

For those in the African American population, the results of the Tuskegee study still linger. This research study, which began in 1932, was facilitated by the U.S. Public Health Service Syphilis Study at Tuskegee, and recruited 600 African American men, 399 with syphilis and 201 without. The goal was to find an effective treatment. It was to have lasted six months; it continued for 40 years. The men were never told specific information, only that they were being treated for "bad blood." They were given free medical exams and free meals, and their burial expenses were paid. Although penicillin, an effective treatment of syphilis became available in 1947, it was not offered to the participants. It was not until 1972, when the Associated Press did a story about the Tuskegee Study, that this information came to light. A public outcry ensued. The study ended in October of 1972 (Center for

Disease Control and Prevention). Mistrust of those in healthcare continues to be a barrier to care and leads to health disparities.

I'd like to share a story about a discussion I had with my sister-in-law, "Susan," last year. My brother-in-law, "James," was diagnosed with lung cancer and was receiving treatment. Susan, an African American and licensed vocational nurse, had worked for more than 30 years at various hospitals in the area. She was able to maneuver through the health system easily, knew the questions that needed to be asked, and was an advocate for James. Yet, as his condition worsened, she became more suspicious and less trusting of the physician and the healthcare personnel. She made sure she went to every visit because, as she shared with me, "You never know what they might try to do to him." Here is a person who is a professional and knowledgeable, but her lived history told her that health personnel may not be trusted to do the right thing for a family member. While it surprised me to hear this, I understood that her story, and her perspective, might that also be the perspective of some of my patients, particularly older patients. And how do I acknowledge this possible unspoken mistrust during the appointment?

Reflective exercise: Trust & Mistrust
1. *Have you ever been in a situation with a HCP where trust was an issue?*
2. *Think of your patients and their histories ~ are there issues of trust?*
3. *In what way could you initiate a dialogue about trust and treatment?*

The bigger picture influences outcomes . . .

Research findings assist the HCP to provide care based on facts and assures, hopefully, a positive health outcome. Until recently, research in the scientific arena has been done primarily on white men. In the article *Ethnic and Racial Health Disparities Research: Issues and Problems* (Sue, Dhindsa 2006), four issues regarding research done with ethnic and gender groups are identified: sampling size (small ethnic/racial population); differences within racial ethnic groups (i.e. Hispanic ~ but cultural beliefs and values may differ between Cuban Americans and Mexican Americans); misunderstanding of questions and possible biased instruments; and financial and/or political support for the study. It took legislation to begin to change those factors. The 1999 Congress requested the Institute of Medicine to:

1. Assess the extent of racial and ethnic disparities in healthcare
2. Identify potential sources of said disparities
3. Suggest intervention strategies

With acknowledgment comes change. Who is addressing these issues of healthcare disparities in ethnic minorities and other vulnerable populations?

What an expert panel had to say . . .

The American Academy of Nursing (AAN) was formed in 1973 by the American Nurses Association and is considered the "think tank of nursing." An invitation-only group, it serves the public and the nursing profession by advancing health policy and practice through the generation, synthesis, and dissemination of nursing knowledge. Recently, they convened a panel with expertise in cultural competence and healthcare. The AAN wanted to "know what the experts know" about culture and health disparities and to solicit recommendations on the subject.

The panel, Drs. Giger, Davidhizar, Purnell, Harden, Phillips, and Strickland, each an expert in the field of cultural diversity and healthcare, provided an excellent overview of the links between cultural competency and health disparities. In the article, *American Academy of Nursing Expert Panel Report: Developing Cultural Competence to Eliminate Health Disparities in Ethnic Minorities and Other Vulnerable Populations* (2007), they state that statistics indicate a higher morbidity and mortality in ethnic minorities and other vulnerable groups. The inclusion of women and minority groups in research ensuring the use of cultural interventions was at the top of the list of recommendations. Others included the areas of education, practice, research, policy, and advocacy. They cite the National Center for Minority Health recommendations, which state that cultural competence can be used to counteract discrepancies in health disparities.

Insights from the Institute of Medicine

In addition to the AAN Expert Panel on Cultural Competence, the Institute of Medicine report of 2003, *Unequal Treatment: Confronting Racial and Ethnic Disparities in Healthcare*, concludes that "the sources of these disparities are complex, are rooted in historic and contemporary inequities, and involve many participants at several levels, including health systems, their administrative and bureaucratic processes, utilization managers, health care professionals and patients" (Nelson et al., p. 1). We are all players in this process, thus each of us must be part of the solution as well. While there are a number of factors, both positive and negative, that can affect health outcomes; some are rooted in conscious and unconscious stereotyping of the patients. Other factors may include trust – mistrust of the HCP, language, time constraints and available resources. As we review each, think about your clinical area and your patients.

Stereotyping seems to always be at the head of the list, and while we as HCP are dedicated to our profession and believe we provide equality to all the persons we care for within our area of expertise, there are still, according to current statistics, differences in health outcomes. It may be easy for us to see our perspective and think we have the correct approach, but that may be quite different from the approach of our patients. Previous encounters with our patients may influence the interaction as well. Acknowledgment of bias is the first step in eliminating disparities.

Reflective exercise: Thoughts on previous experience
1. *Think about a positive encounter with someone different from yourself – what aspects made it that way?*
2. *A negative encounter – what do you think made it that way?*
3. *What would you do differently?*

Navigating the system . . .

We know how to navigate the healthcare system: whom to call, what to ask, and where to find resources. We know the terminology and are comfortable walking into any healthcare arena; even if it is not our area of expertise, we can still converse with the other HCPs in that setting. So, when a member of our family or a good friend is in need of expert healthcare, we can make it happen! But, let's say you needed a "good" lawyer. Would you know whom to call and what questions to ask? Would you "understand" the jargon? If you didn't, would you feel comfortable asking for clarification?

Now let's think about your patients. Do they have the ability to navigate through the system, ask relevant questions, and have the confidence to speak up when there is a lack of understanding? For some patients, seeking healthcare can be an anxiety-producing experience based on prior negative encounters or unfamiliarity with the system. For others, it may include a distrust or mistrust of the system – stories they have heard from others within their family or community. As HCPs, we are called to consider the patient's history, educational level, and language, as well as cultural beliefs and healthcare practices. In what way can we be the bridge that enables the patient to feel welcome? One answer is to acknowledge that disparities exist and to believe that, together with patients, we can create positive outcomes.

Bring up the subject: talk about the uncomfortable, acknowledge the differences, and ask the patient, "What do I need to know from you that will make this meeting and future ones a positive experience?"

Better access to care may be one of the responses from the patient. Clinic location, availability of transportation, and flexible appointments are some elements that may need to be considered. Another important factor is the time allocated for each encounter. Is there enough time during the interview process to gather essential information? Allocating a few minutes more specifically to focus on the patient's expectations related to healthcare may make a difference in outcome. It may also, more importantly, establish the HCP's interest in knowing more about the patient, "the person." Showing a curious and genuine interest creates a comfortable and welcoming environment for both patient and HCP.

Are there the resources available to assist in this process? A resource of "time" may be one factor, but the availability of medication or medical supplies is another. An interesting example of limited resources was highlighted in the article, *Research and Educational Approaches to Reducing Health Disparities among American Indians and Alaska Natives* (Warne 2006). It seems that a "once-a-day" or "long-acting" medication for diabetes is not on the formulary for the Indian Health Services because of cost. The available medication is scheduled two to three times each day. A once-a-day medication regime is more likely to be followed than multi-dose, thus providing improved patient health outcomes.

> **Reflective exercise: From the patient's perspective**
> 1. *How easy is it for your patients to "navigate" through your health facility?*
> 2. *Are you familiar with the cultural beliefs and healthcare practices of your patients?*
> 3. *Are there flexible clinic appointments at your facility?*
> 4. *Is transportation readily available to your patients?*
> 5. *What would you change at your facility to improve access . . . resources?*

Where to from here?

Education is the number one recommendation found throughout the literature: Education for HCPs on the cultural values, beliefs, and healthcare practices of diverse populations and educational material that is culturally appropriate for patients.

Education

- **Expert Panel:** ~ The AAN will collaborate with other organizations to:
  - ☐ Establish ways to teach and guide faculty and nursing students to provide culturally competent nursing care practices to clients in diverse clinical settings.
  - ☐ Promote the development of a document that supports the regulation of content reflecting diversity in nursing curricula.

- **Institute of Medicine:**
  - ☐ Patient ~ improve knowledge of how to access care & participate in clinical decision making.
  - ☐ Healthcare provider ~ provide tools to manage cultural and linguistic diversity of patients, avoid unconscious biases and stereotypes to affect interaction with patient.
  - ☐ Cross-cultural curricula ~ integrate early in training.

Reflective exercise: Education

1. *Have you had the opportunity to discuss influences of history, past and current, on healthcare decisions?*
2. *Does your institution provide educational seminars on the cultural characteristics of ethnic and cultural groups?*
3. *Are there discussions that help you understand the ways in which language and culture may influence healthcare behaviors and practices?*
4. *If so, what are you or your institution doing to narrow and eventually eliminate those disparities?*

Continued Research

Research is vital to reducing and ultimately eliminating poor health outcomes found in minority groups and other vulnerable populations. The elimination of barriers, along with the implementation of a trusting and respectful relationship with the patient and community, helps to ensure a reduction in health disparities. Using this collaborative approach leads to positive interactions. Recommendations found in the article, *Research and Educational Approaches to Reducing Health Disparities among American Indians and Alaskan Native* (2006), provide excellent guidelines to be considered for future research studies.

Recommendations

- **Improved trust** by providing communities a voice in research agenda setting and design
- **Increased benefits** by involving the community in linking results to application through policy development
- **Greater understanding** in the research and academic communities of cultural factors and other issues that lead to health disparities
- **Improved cultural appropriateness** of research design, implementation and characterization of results.

<u>Reflective exercise</u>: **Research**
5. *Think about your patient population ~ where do you see healthcare disparities?*
6. *If given the opportunity to discover ways to eliminate disparities, where would your research be focused?*
7. *How would you disseminate your finding?*
8. *How would you design your program?*
9. *How would you orient it to educate both patients and HCPs?*

Continuing the Journey . . .

Healthcare disparities are a fact. Our job as a HCP is to identify the gaps in care when we see them. We may find them at the registration desk, or they may surface during the assessment phase as pertinent information is gathered about the patient's status. They may come during the physical exam and our knowledge of biological variations found in various ethnic groups. Making that next appointment may seem like a small part, but do we consider the variables of access to transportation, telephone or the literacy level of the patient? Again, if we as HCPs were to put ourselves in another arena, such as a courtroom pleading our case, how much would we know to facilitate a good outcome? Could we "navigate" the systems, would we be familiar with the language of the lawyers? Maybe. But likely not. The fact is that we are in the healthcare arena. We are knowledgeable about the "way it works" and we know the language of medicine. In addition, we must strive to understand the value placed by our patients, consciously or unconsciously, on their cultural beliefs and on our ability to care for them.

Resources

Allison, J. J. (2007). Health disparity: Causes, consequences and change. *Medical Care, Research and Review*. (64)5. 5S-6S.

Andrews, M. M., Boyle, J. S. (2008). *Transcultural concepts in nursing care*. (5th Ed.).New York: Lippincott Williams & Wilkins.

Betancourt, J. R., Green, A. R., Carrillo, J. E., Firempong, O. A. (2003). Defining cultural competence: A practical framework for addressing racial/ethnic disparities in health and health care. *Public Health Reports* July/August. Vol 118. p.293-302.

Center for Disease Control and Prevention. U.S. Public Health Service Syphilis Study at Tuskegee. Retrieved on November 2, 2009, from www.cdc.gov/tuskegee/timeline

Chin, M. H., Walters, A. E., Cook, S. C., Huang, E. S. (2007). Interventions to reduce racial and ethnic disparities in health care. *Medical Care, Research and Review*. (64)5. 7S-28S.

Dayton, E., Zhan, C., Sangl, J., Darby, C., Moy, E. (2006). Racial and ethnic differences in patient assessments of interactions with providers: Disparities or measurement bias. *Journal of Medical Quality*. (21)2. 109114.

Frist, W. H., Landrieu, M. (2004). Closing the health care gap ~ Legislative Summary. Retrieved March 2005 from www.frist.senate.gov

Giger, J. N., Davidhizar, R. E. (2008). *Transcultural nursing: Assessment and intervention*. (5th Ed.). St Louis, MO: Mosby/Elsevier.

Giger, J., Davidhizar, R., Purnell, L., Harden, J., Phillips, J., Stickland. (2007). American Academy of Nursing Expert Panel Report: Developing cultural competence to eliminate health disparities in ethnic minorities and other vulnerable populations. *Journal of Transcultural Nursing*. (18) 2, 95-102.

Grahm-Garcia, J., Raines, T. L., Andrews, J. O., Mensah, G. A. (2001). Race, ethnicity, and geography: Disparities in heart disease in women of color. *Journal of Transcultural Nursing*. (12)1. 56-67.

Leininger, M. M. (1991). *Culture care diversity and universality: A theory of nursing*. New York: National League for Nursing Press.

Leininger, M. M., McFarland, M. R. (2002). *Transcultural nursing: Concepts, theories, research and practice*. (3rd Ed.). New York: McGraw-Hill.

MacNaughton, N. S. (2008). Health disparities and health-seeking behavior among Latino men: A review of the literature. *Journal of Transcultural Nursing*. (19)1.83-91.

Murray, C., Woods, V. D. (2009). Psychology of Health Disparities among African American populations: An overview. *Journal of Black Psychology*. (35)2, 142-145.

National Institute of Health. (2006). Fact sheet: Health disparities. 1-2.

Office of Majority Leader William H. Frist, M.D. (2004). "Closing the health care gap: Legislative Summary. Retrieved on January 6, 2005, from www.frist.senate.gov

Penner, L. A., Dovidio, J. F., Edmondson, D., Dailey, R. K., Markova, T., Albrecht, T., Gaertner, S. (2009). The experience of discrimination and Black-White health disparities in medical care. *Journal of Black Psychology*. 35(2). 180-203.

Purnell, L. D., Paulanka, B. J. (2008). *Transcultural Health Care: A Culturally Competent Approach*. (3rd Ed.). Philadelphia, PA: F. A. Davis Company.

Sisk, J. E., Sonnenfeld, N. (2008). Health care disparities research: Using the National Health Care Surveys. *Center for Disease Control and Preventation*.

Smedley, B., Stith, A., Nelson, A. (2002). Unequal treatment: Confronting racial and ethnic disparities in health care. Institute of Medicine. Washington D.C.: The National Academies Press.

Smith, G. R. (2007). Health disparities: What can nursing do? *Policy, Politics, & Nursing Practice*. (8)4. 285-291.

Spector, R. (2009). *Cultural diversity in health and illness*. (7th Ed.), New Jersey: Pearson/Prentice Hall.

Sue, S., Dhindsa, M. K. (2006). Ethnic and racial health disparities research: Issues and problems. *Health Education & Behavior*. (33)4. 459-469.

Villarruel, A. M. (2007). Poverty and health disparities: More than just a difference. Western Journal of Nursing Research. (29)6, 654-656.

Warne, D. (2006). Research and educational approaches to reducing health disparities among American Indians and Alaska Natives. Journal of Transcultural Nursing. (17)3. 266-271.

U.S. Department of Health and Human Services. (2004). Closing the quality gap: A critical analysis of quality improvement strategies. Agency for Healthcare, Research and Quality. Retrieved on November 14, 2009, from www.ahrq.gov/clinic/epe

U.S. Department of Health and Human Services (2003). National Healthcare Disparities Report of 2003. Agency for Health Care Research. Retrieved September 16, 2010 from www.ahrq.gov

Barriers . . . What Is Getting in the Way?

6

Barriers, while obvious to those outside of the healthcare arena, may be less apparent to those of us who work in the clinical setting. We understand the jargon, the culture, and the ways things are done. It seems routine to us. Yet, think back to your first day on the job. Did you feel out of your element? Did everybody else seem to know what they were doing except you? I remember feeling very inept, asking too many questions (I thought) and wishing it were six months later when all of this would be familiar.

Now, let's think about our patients. For some or most of them, the healthcare world seems daunting as they attempt to maneuver through the system. In this chapter barriers to healthcare are identified. Join us on this journey as seen through the eyes of our patients. But first, a bit of history.

Healthcare reform then and now

Healthcare reform has been in progress for over a hundred years. Each time the issues have been similar: a large number of uninsured people and growing health concerns. Outcomes were the same: healthcare legislation failed to pass. To help understand today's debate about healthcare reform, it is important that we visit the past. In reality it has been at the forefront of many a political discussion since the Healthcare Initiative of President Theodore Roosevelt to the proposal by the Barack Obama administration.

While the Socialist Party had endorsed a compulsory healthcare program in 1904, it was not until 1912 that the Progressive Party candidate Theodore Roosevelt advocated for national health insurance in his party's platform. It said, "We pledge ourselves to work unceasingly in State and Nation for . . . the protection of home life against the hazards of sickness, irregular employment and old age through the adoption of a system of social insurance adapted to American use" (www.socialsecurity.gov/history). Unfortunately, he lost the election.

In the article, *Health Care Reform and Social Movements in the United States* (2002), Beatrix Hoffman, PhD, writes that many of the successful social movements in the 20th century relied on grassroots participation – people advocating for reform. Healthcare reform movements, however, were headed by academics, economists, and organizations; thus, they were minimally successful.

In 1915, the American Association for Labor Legislation, a group of academics, submitted a proposal advocating for health insurance that would protect ill workers against loss of wages and medical costs. This proposal, modeled after programs in Germany and England, received support from the public, but was defeated in Congress. In the 1920s, a group called the Committee on Costs of Medical Care, supported by academics, economists, and physicians, put their confidence in research rather than people. The legislation was defeated.

In 1945, the Wagner-Murray-Dingell Bill was proposed as a national medical insurance program that was to be financed by social security payroll taxes. While it was supported by then president Harry S. Truman, it was defeated as well. It was in July of 1965, during President Lyndon Johnson's term, that Medicare, having been worked on for over a decade, was signed into law. Building on that, Richard Nixon in his address to the Congress in 1971 proposed a National Health Strategy that would address the shortcomings in the healthcare system, including access to care, cost, and availability of healthcare professionals. In 1993, President Bill Clinton initiated discussion on healthcare reform as well. While initially applauded, it was later criticized by congressional members and never got beyond the discussion phase.

That all changed on March 21, 2010, when the House of Representatives passed the Health Care Reform Bill (HR 3590 Patient Protection and Affordable Care Act) that had been submitted to them by the Senate. It was signed into law by President Barack Obama on Tuesday, March 23, 2010. The House amendments, which required Senate approval, were passed on March 25, 2010. What started over a hundred years ago is now law.

As HCPs, we readily acknowledge that we are part of the solution as well. We have the expertise and the experience to ensure patients receive the healthcare they need. Reflect on some of the ways we can open doors and provide care and resources for our patients.

Reflective exercise: Thinking outside the box
1. *In what ways can we increase access to care?*
2. *Are our hours of operation meeting the needs of our patient/patient population?*
3. *Have our interpreters received medical and cultural training?*
4. *Do we involve the community in our decision-making process?*
5. *Does our educational material meet the learning needs of our patients?*
6. *Does our staff reflect the diversity of our patient population?*

In addition to insurance, other compelling issues that affect access to care include language, education, literacy, acculturation, and availability of bilingual and bicultural healthcare professionals. Recognition of the need and a desire for change are the first steps in the process. In the next section we review each issue and identify ways to eliminate these barriers to our patients.

Socioeconomic

Facts are important and set the stage for understanding the magnitude of living in a world in which money and/or income dictates one's ability to meet even the basic needs. Socioeconomics has always played a role in healthcare, as noted in the healthcare reform section. According to the U.S. Census Report issued in September 2010, the median income is now $49,777. The range of income varies from a low of $32,584 for African Americans to a high of $65,469 for Asians. Regionally, the West has the highest median household income of $53,833, followed by the Northeast and Midwest with the South having the lowest income of $45,615. Women make 77 cents on every dollar a man makes. There continue to be economic discrepancies between gender, race, and region. This impacts the ability to pay for healthcare.

There are over 37 million people living in poverty in the United States. While that may be only 10% of the total population, it still remains that 37 million people wake up to that fact each day. According to the U.S. Census Bureau Report of 2007, the change from the previous census was "not statistically significant." Those who live with poverty every day would probably put more emphasis on the word "significant." While other aspects of their life may be within their power to control, finances are not. Let's look more closely at those who live at or below the poverty level.

Poverty in the United States

American Indian	24.2%
African American	25.8%
Hispanic	25.3%
Asian	12.5%
White	9.4%

Cite: U.S. Census Bureau 2010

Currently for a family of four, the United States poverty level is set at $21,203, up from $19,971 in 2005. Dividing that by twelve months leaves the family with $1767 per month or $60 per day to cover rent, utilities, food, transportation, clothing, and healthcare needs. As HCPs we can easily see that there may be no money left to purchase medication or pay out of pocket for medical services, let alone get to and from clinic appointments.

<u>Reflective exercise</u>: **Socioeconomics**
1. *Have you experienced poverty?*
2. *What are the socioeconomic demographics of your patient population?*
3. *How does your patient population compare/contrast with you?*
4. *What are some of the ways you can ensure access to care?*

Health Insurance

Is health insurance the key to wellness? Maybe. Having health insurance makes it possible to seek care, get diagnostic testing, receive physical and/or occupational therapy, get mental health counseling, receive home health visits, and pay for medications . . . right? Maybe not. Services are dependent on the type of coverage and are affected by deductibles, co-pay and which providers accept your insurance. If finances are an issue, then the choice of coverage is based primarily on cost. For some patients, paying $500 or $1,500 per month for health insurance can be the difference between putting food on the table for their family and going hungry. For the working poor, those who work yet are unable to pay for insurance, the likelihood of securing insurance is questionable.

"Premiums Rise 5% for a Year: Increase is 131% for Decade" was the headline story recently in the San Francisco Chronicle (2010). The report by the Kaiser Family Foundation and Health Research and Educational Trust comes at a crucial time. It reports that while there was a 131% increase in health care premiums, wages increased only by 38%.

According to the U.S. Census Bureau (2007), 27% of persons are covered by government insurance (Medicare, Medicaid, Military healthcare, State Children's Health Insurance Program and individual state health plans), while 68% are covered by private insurance (plans provided by employers or a union or purchased by an individual from a private company).

Let's look specifically at the uninsured from the point of ethnicity, age, and household income. Think about your patient population as you review these statistics posted by the U.S. Census Bureau report, *Income, Poverty and Health Insurance coverage in the United States: 2009.*

Uninsured by Ethnicity

32.4%	Hispanic
31.7%	American Indian
21%	African American
17.2%	Asian American
12%	White, non-Hispanic

Uninsured by Age

10%	Under 18 years
30.4%	18-24 years
29.1%	25-34 years
21.7%	35-44 years
16.1%	45-64 years
1.8%	65 years and older

Uninsured by Household Income

26.2%	less than $25,000
21.4%	$25,000 – 49, 999
16%	$50,000 – 74, 999
9%	$75,000 or more

Reflective exercise: Health Insurance
1. *Have you ever gone without health insurance?*
2. *What was your greatest concern or fear during that time?*
3. *Think about your patient population ~ what percent are uninsured?*
4. *What resources are in place within your organization to meet these needs?*

Language

Language is how one communicates needs and gains knowledge. Persons not fluent in English may hesitate to seek care unless translators are available. Numerous studies have shown that those who do not speak English are less likely to receive the same treatment as those who do. According to the United States Census Bureau (2000), nearly 14 million Americans are not proficient in English. The *2007 American Community Survey* (2007) indicates that more than 19.7%, or nearly fifty million people, speak a language other than English at home. That number is an increase over the past decade.

Language Use and English Speaking Ability: 2000 issued in 2003 by the U.S. Census Bureau indicates that there are more than 380 categories of single languages spoken by the persons living in the United States. Those households deemed *linguistically isolated* are defined as those in which no one over the age of 14 speaks English at least "very well." The 2000 census showed an increase in this category from 2.9 million households in 1990 to 4.4 million in 2000.

Those who spoke English "less than well" were found predominately in Florida, California and Texas. The fewest were found in the Midwest. But, as HCPs, we know that statistics are just that – statistics – and are not reflective of your site. Lack of bilingual/bicultural HCPs may be perceived by your patients as a barrier to care.

**Speakers of Language Other Than English at Home
and English Ability by Languge Group: 2000**

(Population 5 years and over, in millions. Data based on sample. For information on confidentiality protection, nonsampling error, sampling error, and definitions, see www.census.gov/prod/cen2000/doc/sf3.pdf)

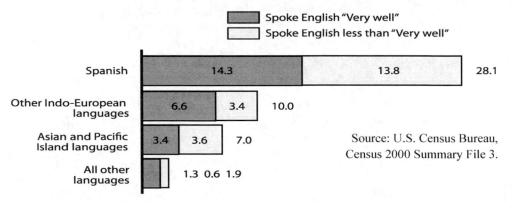

Figure 6-1-A: Lanuages Spoken

Ten Languages Most Frequently Spoken at Home Other Than English and Spanish: 2000

(Population 5 years and over, in millions. Data based on sample. For information on confidentiality protection, nonsampling error, sampling error, and definitions, see www.census.gov/prod/cen2000/doc/sf3.pdf)

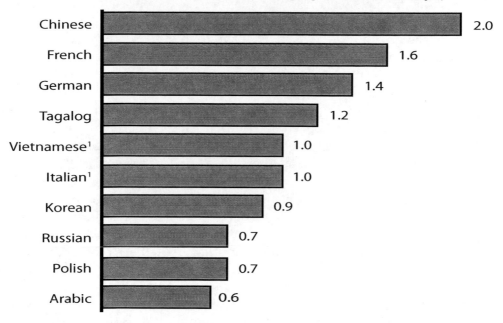

Chinese	2.0
French	1.6
German	1.4
Tagalog	1.2
Vietnamese[1]	1.0
Italian[1]	1.0
Korean	0.9
Russian	0.7
Polish	0.7
Arabic	0.6

[1]The number of Vietnamese speakers and the number of Italian speakers were not statistically different from one another.
Note: The estimates in this figure vary from actual values due to samplng errors. As a result, the number of speakers of some languages shown in this figure may not be statistically different from the number of speakers of languages not shown in this figure.

Source: U.S. Census Bureau, Census 2000 Summary File 3.

Figure 6-1-B: Lanuages Spoken

Lost in translation . . . ?

As HCPs we face the challenge of language on a daily basis. Ideally, there are health professionals on staff within the organization who speak the patient's language and understand the culture. However, we frequently rely on nonprofessional staff or family members to translate. In either case, unless an interpreter training program is in place, there is minimal assurance that medical information is translated effectively to the patient. Furthermore, asking a family member to translate does not always ensure accuracy.

The patient may choose not to share information pertinent to the case because they do not want the family to know personal issues. The HCP, in turn, may not get the whole story.

There are some basic principles to follow when using an interpreter. First, you should meet with the interpreter prior to the encounter and discuss the information you need to share with the patient. It is vital that the entire response made by the patient is given. The following example exemplifies the importance of interpreting all the information shared A question is asked of the patient, "What time do you take your medication each day?" The response may go on for several minutes, after which time the interpreter says to you, "about 7:00 p.m." Two thoughts emerge – one from you and one from the patient. The patient may think that the interpreter did not tell the whole story; thus, trust could become an issue. The HCP may come to the same conclusion – what information was not shared? For many cultural groups, it is in "sharing the story," that the message is encoded. The patient may have shared that she gets up in the morning, does not take the medication because it upsets her stomach and makes her dizzy, and that is why she waits until the end of the day. A person trained in medical translation would acknowledge the importance of that information and provide the HCP with the whole story.

Beyond words, messages are communicated through body language and tone of voice. According to Dr. Mehrabin (1969), 55% of what we say is body language, 38% is tone of voice, and only 7% is words. Here are some additional suggestions to ensure understanding. First, always look at the patient when asking the question, and continue to observe during the translation period. What is her body language and tone of voice saying?

> **Reflective exercise: Language**
> 1. *Have you ever been traveling in a foreign country, gotten sick and sought medical care?*
> 2. *How did you get your message across to the HCP in that situation?*
> 3. *What is the predominate language of your patients spoken at your site?*
> 4. *Do you speak another language? If not, which one would you like to learn?*
> 5. *Is there a translator class offered by your organization?*
> 6. *What percentage of HCPs is bilingual and bicultural?*

Think about the community you serve and the languages spoken. What resources are available to you to learn another language? Are classes offered through your community college or within your organization? An additional resource is immersion programs. These programs are found in many different countries and offer daily language classes and housing with a host family. Language skills and cultural knowledge are the dividends of immersion programs. An even greater reward is the smile on your patient's face when you speak and they understand.

Education level . . . Literacy level

The key to reaching across the divide between HCP and patient in addition to communication skills is education and the patient's ability to read and understand handouts. Literacy, as defined as the ability to read and write, may or may not correlate with a patient's educational level. According to the National Assessment of Adult Literacy (2006), more that 14% of the population is below basic in health literacy. Eight million persons cannot read the label: *"Keep out of reach of children!"* That's eye opening!

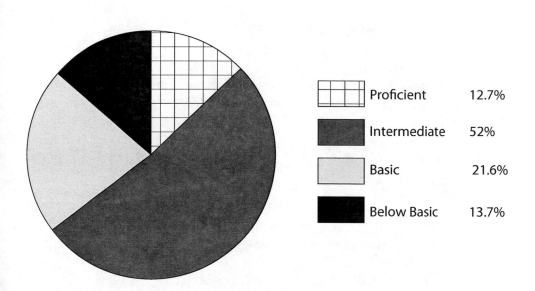

Proficient	12.7%
Intermediate	52%
Basic	21.6%
Below Basic	13.7%

Figure 6-2: Health Literacy

Definitions:

<u>**Proficient**</u>: can perform **complex** literacy activities

<u>**Intermediate**</u>: can perform **moderately** challenging literacy activities

<u>**Basic**</u>: can perform **simple** everyday tasks

<u>**Below basic**</u>: can perform **no more than the simplest** and concrete literacy activity

The assessment survey indicates that White and Asian/Pacific Islander adults have a higher health literacy level than Black, Hispanic, American Indian/Alaskan Native and multiracial adults. Reflect for a moment on the educational material available within your department – the handouts, brochures, and instructional sheets. Do they match your patient's literacy level?

Health education material, according to *The Institute of Medicine of the National Academics Health Literacy* (2004), generally is written at the eighth to ninth grade level, hospital consent forms at the college level. For a large portion of persons residing in the United States who are at the basic level and below, it may be a daunting task to read and understand the contents. Health education material should reflect the population of the community, taking into account the education and literacy level and the culture.

Here are some suggestions:

- Written material should have large amounts of white space so as to appear uncluttered, have large type set (12 pt or more) and good illustrations that reflect the written information.
- Age, gender and culture must be considered in the design of the material.
- Translation of the material into another language takes additional focus requiring two or more native speakers to back-translate the material and ensure understanding.
- Clip art needs to be sensitive to the cultural group as well.
- Personalize the information by using the word "you."
- Medical terminology that would not be understood by the patient should be avoided.
- The document should have good readability.

Another tool for establishing rapport and trust

Neurolinguistic Programming (NLP) is an excellent way to eliminate barriers, establish rapport, and build trust. It is a style of communication based on the way we take in information, encode it, and use it to convey our message. Information is received through our five senses: sight, sound, feeling, smell, and taste. One or two of these are usually dominant. For example, if you were describing a parade and you encode using sight, your response includes colors, float designs and costumes worn by the participants. If you are auditory, you talk about the sounds you heard. Listen to your patients' words as they tell you about the current health concern. Are they visual, auditory, feeling, taste, or smell? Now, using this information, begin to ask questions. If your patient is an auditory person, you would ask "what sound did you hear when you twisted your ankle?" In this way the patient describes the health issue the way she encodes information. You will find that you will gather more information about their condition by using this technique.

Reflective exercise: Education and Literacy
1. *What is the literacy level of our patient population?*
2. *Does our educational material match the literacy level of our patients?*
3. *How do you encode and take in information?*

Acculturation and Language

There are a variety of viewpoints and strong opinions about immigrants learning English and assimilating into the American culture. Acculturation or assimilation may factor into one's ability to access healthcare. In a poll conducted by the Pew Research Center in 2006, 44% of Americans believed that the immigrants of today are not as willing to assimilate as those who came in the early 20th century. For some this may be true. Acculturation may be the first thought and focus of a new immigrant or may not occur until the second or third generation. In his article, *Engine of Assimilation – the Economy* (2008), Tomas Jimenez, an assistant professor of sociology at UC San Diego, suggests that assimilation is not a choice, but rather a direct relationship with the opportunity to improve one's economic and educational position.

As HCPs who care for multi-ethnic and multi-generational populations, we need to view each person as a unique individual and not categorize each based on their level of perceived assimilation to this country. Remember how it feels to be new . . . the new employee . . . the new student, or the new kid in the neighborhood? All things are uncomfortable and uncertain. Consider the newly arrived immigrants and those who have lived here for twenty years. Think of ways to promote understanding, and to create a welcoming environment.

Bilingual/Bicultural Providers

You walk into the hospital or clinic or outpatient therapy department – does anyone look like you or talk like you? If the answer is yes, then there is a sense of familiarity and assurance. But what if no one matches you? Would you still feel that level of comfort and familiarity? Perhaps not. Think about your patient population and your staff population. Do they match? And really, is that important? In one study involving African American patients and White providers, it was noted that the trust level between the patient and the providers was less than that of the other groups.

Current demographics show an increase in ethnic diversity of nurses, social workers, and physicians over the past decade. Given that the current U.S. population is significantly more diverse than HCPs, outreach programs to encourage minority students to enter into the healthcare profession are vital. This concept is recognized by many in the health profession, in academia, and in the United States Congress. In *Closing the Health Care Gap Act 2004*, as previously mentioned in Chapter 3, "Demographics," identified educational and recruitment of minority groups as essential to the elimination of barriers to care and increased access to care. Here are their recommendations.

Professional Education, Awareness and Training

- Workforce Diversity and Training
  - ☐ Increase underrepresented minority students and faculty
  - ☐ Provide funds for scholarships
  - ☐ Increase individuals from disadvantaged backgrounds
- Increase flexibility for use of Higher Education Act funds for historically Black Graduate Institutions
- Model Cultural Competency Curriculum Development
  - ☐ Demonstrate series to test models curricula
  - ☐ Identify barriers to culturally appropriate care
  - ☐ Implement online library with clinically relevant cultural information

The 2002 report by the IOM, *Unequal Treatment: What Health Care System Administrators Need to Know about Racial and Ethnic Disparities in Healthcare*, suggests that both patient and HCPs could benefit from culturally appropriate education. Providing on-site cultural awareness education seminars for staff increases the cultural knowledge and skills necessary to provide culturally competent health to a diverse population. Providing patients with information about ways to access healthcare, to participate in decision making with the HCP and to navigate the health care system may increase their confidence to advocate for their needs. Together with our patients we can address issues and work collaboratively to eliminate the barriers to healthcare.

Resources

Andrews, M. M., Boyle, J. S. (2008). *Transcultural concepts in nursing care*. (5th Ed.).New York: Lippincott Williams & Wilkins.

Campinha-Bacote, J. (2003). The process of cultural competence in the delivery of healthcare services: A culturally competent model of care. Cincinnati, OH: Transcultural C.A.R.E. Associates.

Farrell, C. (2006). It's time to cure health care. *Business Week*. www.businessweek.com

Giger, J. N., Davidhizar, R. E. (2008). Transcultural nursing: Assessment and intervention. (5th Ed.). St Louis, MO: Mosby/Elsevier.

Giger, J. N., Davidhizar, R., Purnell, L., Harden, J., Phillips, J., Stickland. (2007). American Academy of Nursing Expert Panel Report: Developing cultural competence to eliminate health disparities in ethnic minorities and other vulnerable populations. *Journal of Transcultural Nursing*. (18) 2, 95-102.

Hoffman, B. (2003). Health Care Reform and Social Movements in the United States. *American Journal of Public Health*. (93)1. 75-85.

Institute of Medicine of the National Academics. (2004). Health Literacy: A prescription to end confusion. Retrieved on July 9, 2009 from www.iom/edu

Jimenez, T. R. (2008). Engine of assimilaton – the economy. *San Francisco Chronicle*.

Kaiser Family Foundation. (2009). Focus on health reform: Side by side comparison major health care reform proposals.

Leininger, M. M. (1991). Culture care diversity and universality: A theory of nursing. New York: National League for Nursing Press.

Leininger, M. M., McFarland, M. R. (2002). Transcultural nursing: Concepts, theories, research and practice. (3rd Ed.). New York: McGraw-Hill.

Lipson, J., Dibble, S., (2005). Culture & Clinical Care. San Francisco, CA: UCSF NursingPress

McGoldrick, M, Giordano, J., Garcia-Preto, N. (2005). *Ethnicity & Family Therapy*. (3rd Ed.). New York: Guilford Press

Mehrabin, A. Mehrabin Communication Study 1969. Retrieved November 3, 2009, from www.kaaj/com/psych

Murray, C., Woods, V. D. (2009). Psychology of Health Disparities among African American populations: An overview. *Journal of Black Psychology*. (35)2, 142-145.

Purnell, L. D., Paulanka, B. J. (2008). Transcultural Health Care: A Culturally Competent Approach. (3rd Ed.). Philadelphia, PA: F. A. Davis Company.

Sandoval, V. A., Adams, S. H. (2001). Subtle skills for building rapport using neuro-linguistic programming in the interview room. *FBI Law Enforcement Bulletin* 1-5.

Siatkowshi, A. A. (2007). Hispanic acculturation: A concept analysis. *Journal of Transcultural Nursing*. (18)4, 316-323.

Smedley, B., Stith, A., Nelson, A. (2002). Unequal treatment: Confronting racial and ethnic disparities in health care. Institute of Medicine. Washington D.C.: The National Academies Press.

Spector, R. (2009). *Cultural diversity in health and illness*. (7th Ed.), New Jersey: Pearson/Prentice Hall.

University of Kentucky. (2009). Cross-Cultural Communication. Office of Student Activities, Leadership & Involvement. www.uky.edu/studentactivities/leadership

U.S. Census Bureau (2010). Income, Poverty and health Insurance Coverage in the United States: 2009. Retrieved September 16, 2010, from www.census.gov

U.S. Census Bureau. (2003). Language use and English-speaking ability: 2000. U.S. Department of Commerce: Economics and Statistics Administration.

U.S. Department of Education. (2003). A first look at the literacy of America's adults in the 21st century. National Center for Educational Statistics.

U.S. Department of Education. (2003). Institute of Education Sciences. National Center for Education Statistics. A first look at the literacy of America's adults in the 21st century. NCES 2006-470.

U.S. Department of Social Security. (2003). Social Insurance Movement. Retrieved March 8, 2010, from www.socialsecurity.gov/history

Villarruel, A. M. (2007). Poverty and health disparities: More than just a difference. *Western Journal of Nursing Research*. (29)6, 654-656.

Wooley, J. T., Peters, G. (2009). The American Presidency Report. University of California: Santa Barbara.

Culture Care Theory . . . Putting It into Practice | 7

"The goal is to provide culturally congruent care that is beneficial, will fit with and is useful to the client, family or cultural group healthy lifeways."

– Dr. Madeleine Leininger

Early on in her career, Dr. Madeleine Leininger had an experience that would change the course of events of her life. In the mid-1950s, while working at a psychiatric facility for disturbed children from various ethnic groups, she realized that the same mode of care given to each child did not produce similar results. In her book, *Culture Care Diversity and Universality: A Theory of Nursing* (1991), she shares her "aha" moment: "In a way, I experienced culture shock and I felt helpless to assist children who so clearly expressed different cultural patterns and ways . . . related to playing, sleeping, interaction . . . I was unable to respond appropriately to them. I did not understand their behavior." (p. 14). Dr. Leininger was so moved by that experience that she obtained her PhD in Anthropology, developed the Culture Care Theory, and established transcultural nursing courses at colleges throughout the United States.

In 1974 she created the Transcultural Nursing Society, which publishes the *Journal of Transcultural Nursing* and provides certification in transcultural nursing. This is a woman with a passion and a vision who continues to be a voice for the inclusion of cultural beliefs, values, and healthcare practices in every plan of care.

Culture Care Theory . . . Diversity and Universality

What is theory and why do we need it? Theory along with research provides evidenced-based practice for patient care. The purpose of Dr. Leininger's Theory of Culture Care Diversity and Universality is to discover those common and diverse aspects of various cultural groups, and then to incorporated this information into a culturally competent and sensitive plan of care. Universality refers to those commonalities between and among cultural groups, while diversity highlights the variations and differences. As HCPs we tend to group everyone as "all the same." The reality is that we are looking through our cultural lens. Patients may not see themselves in the context of a specific group either. At a recent seminar one attendee, a Mexican-American, took issue with the cultural beliefs, values, and practices listed for Mexican-Americans. He stated, "Our family isn't like that at all." He was right: there is more diversity within a group than between groups. Differences may include age, socioeconomic status, gender, religious beliefs, or other elements that influence world view.

The goal of Culture Care Diversity and Universality Theory is to "provide culturally congruent care that is beneficial, will fit with and is useful to the client, family or cultural group healthy lifeways." (Leininger, McFarland 2004 p. 39). The most important message – culturally congruent care – is realized when the HCP is knowledgeable about the cultural beliefs, values, and healthcare practices of that group. Highlighted are four of the twelve premises that support the Dr. Leininger's position, tenets, and hunches.

Assumptive Premises of the Theory

* Culturally based care (caring) is essential for well-being, health, growth, survival, and to face handicaps or death

* Culturally based care is the most comprehensive and holistic means to know, explain, interpret, and predict nursing care phenomena and to guide nursing decisions and actions

* Culture care values, beliefs and practices are influenced by and tend to be embedded in the worldview, language, philosophy, religion & spirituality, kinship, social, political, legal, educational, economic, technological, ethnohistorical, and environmental context of cultures

70

* Culturally congruent care and beneficial nursing care can only occur when care values, expressions, or patterns are known and used explicitly for appropriate, safe, and meaningful care

Leininger 1991, p. 79

So herein lies the challenge. While we may not have the time to do extensive reading about the beliefs, values, and practices of various groups, we can ask our patients about their ways of dealing with healthcare. Acknowledgment and appreciation of our query can lead to vital information necessary to provide culturally competent and sensitive healthcare.

Sunrise Delivery Model . . . our guide to understanding

The Sunrise Delivery Model (Figure 7-1), designed by Dr. Leininger, guides the HCP to discover the cultural meanings, patterns, and practices of specific groups. Using a holistic approach, the model takes into account the influence of the patient's worldviews, including cultural and social factors. As the HCP develops a plan of care, consideration must be taken to incorporate the generic or folk healthcare practices of the patient. Realizing that family members may be influential and helpful in this process, the HCP needs to consider them in the decision-making process and plan of care.* The model culminates with transcultural care decisions and actions and includes three modes: preservation, accommodation, and repatterning.

As we go through the model from beginning to end, think about your beliefs, values, and health practices and those of your patients. Acknowledging similarities and differences helps us to find common ground in which to provide culturally competent and sensitive healthcare.

*Health Insurance Portability and Accountability Act of 1996 (HIPAA) requires that the patient/client must first give permission to disclose any information with family or other individuals.

71

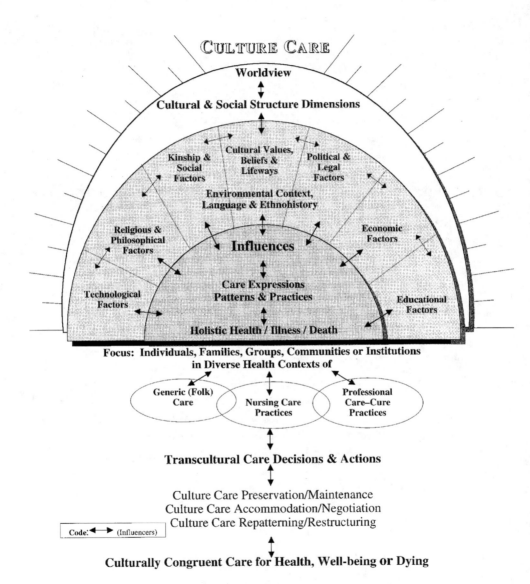

Figure 7-1: Leininger's Sunrise Delivery Model
Reproduced with permission from McGraw Hill Companies.
Transcultural Nursing. ©2003 M. Leininger and M. McFarland.

Worldview

We begin with worldview. How do you "see" the world around you? Who is part of your world and how have they influenced your beliefs, values, and healthcare practices? How is your worldview the same as or different from your patient's? Asking questions of our patients and listening to their responses provides insight and thus an opportunity to see the world from a vantage point that is unknown to us. It is with each successive encounter that acceptance, trust, and respect are established and more information is forthcoming with which to provide quality care.

Worldview inquiries:
- Tell me something about your family of origin.
- Where were your parents born?
- What language is spoken at home?
- What do you like best about your life ~ your world?
- How would you change it?

This is the entry point of the journey – to understand our patients' perspectives of their world. As we review the cultural and social structure dimensions, think about your patient population. The information that we gather from our patients helps to assure a plan of care that, as Dr. Leininger (1991) says, "is beneficial, will fit with and is useful to the patient or family." (p. 13).

Cultural and Social Structure Dimensions

This section of the Sunrise Delivery Model provides the HCP with information that is central to the patient's viewpoint. The process of performing a cultural health assessment provides a holistic picture of the patient or family in which the HCP can discover new information or confirm previous knowledge. Each section offers an insight to our patients' cultural ways of living in the world. It may be helpful to give some examples to the patient prior to each question.

Cultural values, beliefs & lifeways are learned at an early age from our family of origin, extended family, and people we encounter, such as teachers, religious leaders, and healthcare providers. These beliefs and values, held to be true, guide practices and decision making during illness, disease, or death. Conflict can occur when the beliefs and values of the HCP differ from those of the patient. For example, avoiding eye contact during a conversation may be seen as disinterest by the HCP, yet from the patient's point of view, minimal eye contact could be a sign of respect. What do we need to know? Here are some questions that may assist in learning more from the patient:

> **Questions to ask:**
> • What are two important values or beliefs you learned as a child?
> • Who did you learn them from?
> • How do these values and beliefs help you during times of stress, illness, or when facing adversity?

Kinship and Social factors focus on family, extended family, and social organizations. Families may be nuclear or extended. Roles and responsibilities are clearly defined in some families, while others are more egalitarian. Each provide support and care but in different ways. The patient holds beliefs about the role of the sick person and expectations of care from family members during times of illness. Conflict may arise when family members provide total care for the sick person, while the HCP believes that self care assures a speedy recovery. Finding a common ground that values both perspectives ensures good outcomes.

> **Questions to ask:**
> • What are roles and responsibilities of persons in your family?
> • What is the role of the sick person?
> • Who are the caregivers in your family?
> • How are decisions made in your family?

Religion and philosophical factors influence the way one views and finds strength and support during times of illness, disability, or death. Specific rituals such as lighting candles, praying, or reading from of the Qur'an, Bible, Torah, or Book of Mormon may be relied upon during times of uncertainty, providing hope for the patient and family. Other beliefs include wearing strings around the wrist (Hmong) or tying pins to clothing to ensure protection from harm or evil spirits.

> **Questions to ask:**
> • In what ways do your religious/spiritual beliefs and practices help you during uncertain health times?
> • Are there certain rituals that provide comfort and support?
> • If hospitalized, would a visit from your spiritual or religious leader be helpful?

Technological factors are certainly more relevant today that when the model was first developed. The use of cell phones, palm pilots, and computers is integral to many patients' daily lives. Some of my patients have obtained information on the internet which is, in my opinion, a fantastic opportunity to show interest in the patient's resourcefulness and to review this new-found information. Many hospitals and clinics are going paperless, offering patients the opportunity to view lab results, make appointments, and to correspond with their HCP via e-mail.

Questions to ask:
- In what way does this new technological age keep you informed and connected?
- Do you use the internet to learn about health issues?
- In your "every day" ~ is it important to stay connected to family and friends via cell phone? E-mail? Texting?
- What is the best way for the HCP to contact you with test results?

Economic factors, especially in today's world, play an important role in healthcare and treatment. The patient may not be able to follow through with the plan of care due to an unstable economic situation at home. Offering alternatives, providing resources, and taking time to listen can turn a barrier into a bridge. A patient's financial well-being may be a sensitive discussion, but it is vital that the information is available to the HCP to ensure good health outcomes.

Questions to ask:
- Do you need money to maintain your health?
- Have you ever decided not to fill a prescription because you did not have the money?
- Have you gone without health insurance . . . what were your thoughts and concerns during that time?

Political and legal factors affect the patient's ability to obtain and to access healthcare. Insurance companies and/or limited insurance coverage may determine whether a patient receives treatment, pharmaceuticals, or laboratory procedures. In order for the HCP to be the voice for the patient, we must assess their needs and provide information and resources that will help them during times of illness, disability, and death.

Questions to ask:
- Do our laws affect your ability to access healthcare?
- If you could change or add something that would help people stay healthy, what would that be?
- Legally, do you know your rights with regard to healthcare and access?

Educational factors make up one of the most important components of the Sunrise Delivery Model. This section relates to the ability of the patient to read, write, and understand the information relevant to the plan of care. Education is more than a grade level attained; it includes the ways a person learns. Some prefer storytelling, others the internet, and yet another individual might learn best by doing. A variety of teaching modes enable the patient to understand and follow a treatment plan that ensures good outcomes. Here are questions you can ask your patients.

Questions to ask:
- How do you learn best ~ visually, auditory, or hands on?
- Do you prefer a group setting or by yourself?
- Is there a family member you would like to accompany you during a health educational session?
- Can you read and understand handouts and brochures?

Environmental context, Language and Ethnohistory comprise the remaining elements that embrace and influence the patient's view and decisions about health. It is the confluence of both the sociocultural and physical environment: how history, culture, and language are integrated into one's beliefs, values, and health practices. This information, as part of a plan of care, has the most impact on health outcome. It is another opportunity for the HCP to show respect for the patient's culture and to establish rapport.

Questions to ask:
- What are some of the aspects of your culture that you think are the most important with regard to health and illness?
- What language is spoken in your home?
- How would you like to be addressed?
- How should we address your parents? grandparents?

Folk and Generic Practices

The HCP must also take into account the folk or generic care and professional care. Professional care, taught at colleges and universities, promotes a scientific basis for diagnosis, treatment, and cure. Generic or folk practices are traditional ways of healing, and may use indigenous healers to "diagnose and cure." The HCP is trained and knowledgeable about the professional scientific approach to care, while the patient's belief is rooted in folk care. Conflict occurs when a patient believes a folk treatment is effective and the HCP deems it unsafe. Actually this is a great opportunity to dialogue with the patients to discover more about their health practices and beliefs.

Questions to ask:
- What are your beliefs about this illness . . . what do you need to restore your health?
- Did the folk remedy provide the results you expected?
- Do you have concerns about the folk treatment?

Transcultural Care Decisions and Actions

Dr. Leininger presents three modes of care decisions and actions. In each of the preceding sections we gained patient information. Each response is deeply embedded in the patient's belief system; and our mission as HCPs is to listen, learn, and respect the information. During discussions with patients we must consider the impact, positive or negative, of their cultural health beliefs and practices. In some cases these beliefs are preserved and maintained; in others, accommodation or negotiation needs to take place. If the practice poses a threat to the health and wellbeing of the individual, then working collaboratively with the patient to repattern and restructure is required. Think about encounters you have had with patients. What worked and what would you change now that you know?

Preservation/Maintenance is a mode of care in which beliefs and health practices that are valued by the patient are maintained. The HCP can facilitate this by being aware of the cultural beliefs, values, and healthcare practices of the patient and ensuring that these continue to be part of the health plan. Possible healthcare practices might include:

- A string tied around wrist or ankle to protect wellbeing
- Respect for the elderly
- Avoiding eye contact and not raising one's voice
- Praying five times each day
- Visits by a priest, monks, an imam, church elders, deacons

Accommodation/Negotiation is a care mode that assures the patient that the HCP understands these values and makes adjustments to incorporate them into the plan of care. Acknowledgment of the importance of the cultural values demonstrates to the patient an awareness and a respect on the part of the HCP.

These might include:

- Family participation in care
- Obligation and expectation to visit the sick ~ flexible visiting hours
- Kosher meals for the Orthodox Jewish patient
- Ceremonies/rituals in the hospital room for the dying patient
- Overnight accommodation for a parent to stay with a child

Repatterning/Restructuring needs to occur when the current treatment plan that the client is using may be detrimental to health and wellbeing. This may cause tension between the HCP and the client, but it does provide an opportunity for discussion that will hopefully lead to a greater understanding. Collaborating in a respectful manner opens doors to understanding for both parties. Areas where conflict might arise include concepts such as:

- Avoiding surgery until the full moon
- Taking medication only when symptoms are present ~ HTN, NIDM
- Eating large amounts of rice ~ a diabetic client
- Sedentary lifestyle in an obese patient
- Eating for two ~ pregnant woman with gestational diabetes

Dr. Leininger's Culture Care Diversity and Universality Theory and Sunrise Delivery Model offer the HCP a way to gain knowledge about the cultural health practices and the tools to provide care that "fits with and is beneficial and useful to the client and family." Knowledge leads to understanding and understanding to acceptance and respect for differences. The goal is to provide quality care that integrates culture into the plan of care. Culturally competent care is the result of both cultural awareness and knowledge. It is a journey. It begins anew every day.

Resources

Andrews, M. M., Boyle, J. S. (2008). *Transcultural concepts in nursing care*. (5th Ed.).New York: Lippincott Williams & Wilkins.

Campinha-Bacote, J. (2003). The process of cultural competence in the delivery of healthcare services: A culturally competent model of care. Cincinnati, OH: Transcultural C.A.R.E. Associates.

Giger, J. N., Davidhizar, R. E. (2008). *Transcultural nursing: Assessment and Intervention*. (5th Ed.). New York: Mosby.

Giger, J., Davidhizar, R., Purnell, L., Harden, J., Phillips, J., Stickland. (2007). American Academy of Nursing Expert Panel Report: Developing cultural competence to eliminate health disparities in ethnic minorities and other vulnerable populations. *Journal of Transcultural Nursing*. (18) 2, 95-102.

Leininger, M. M. (1989). Transcultural nurse specialist and generalists: New practitioners in nursing. *Journal of Transcultural Nursing*. (1)13. 135-143.

Leininger, M. M. (1991). Culture care diversity and universality: A theory of nursing. New York: National League for Nursing Press.

Leininger, M. M. (1997). Alternative to what? Generic vs professional caring, treatment and healing modes. *Journal of Transcultural Nursing*. (9)1. 37.

Leininger, M. M. (1997). Overview of the Theory of Cultural Care with Ethnonursing research method. *Journal of Transcultural Nursing*. (8)1. 32-52.

Leininger, M. M. (1999). What is transcultural nursing and culturally competent care? *Journal of Transcultural Nursing*. (10)1, p. 9.

Leininger, M. M. (1995). Transcultural nursing: Concepts, theories, research and practice. (2nd Ed.). New York: McGraw-Hill.

Leininger, M. M., McFarland, M. R. (2002). Transcultural nursing: Concepts, theories, research and practice. (3rd Ed.). New York: McGraw-Hill

Lipson, J., Dibble, S., (2005). Culture & Clinical Care (8th Ed.) San Francisco, CA: UCSF NursingPress.

Purnell, L. D., Paulanka, B. J. (2008). Transcultural Health Care: A Culturally Competent Approach. (3rd Ed.). Philadelphia, PA: F. A. Davis Company.

Spector, R. (2009). *Cultural diversity in health and illness*. (7th Ed.), New Jersey: Pearson/Prentice Hall.

Cultural Awareness . . . Humility . . . Competency - Let The Journey Begin!

8

"Culture is a mediator between human beings and chaos, guiding our interactions with each other."

– Julie Lipson 1996

The road to cultural competence begins with "aha" moments of discovery. We suddenly and unexpectedly grasp an understanding of our culture – beliefs, values, and biases – and the ways it guides our interactions, influences our decisions. During those moments we realize our similarities and differences with patients and colleagues. Our willingness to meet and honor those who may be different from us is the beginning of cultural competence. Stops along the way open the door to finding common ground, understanding, and respect.

Culture ~ First Stop

Culture – we all have it. It is how we reveal ourselves. We may not realize its influence because it is so embedded that we take it for granted. However, others may see us differently. Why? Because they view us through their cultural lenses. For those of us working with multi-ethnic communities this could pose a significant dilemma, as our culture may be different from theirs. So how do we bridge this potential barrier? Initially we can start with the understanding that each of us has a culture.

Culture can be defined as beliefs and values passed down from one generation to the next that we hold to be true. Think back to your family of origin. What were the important values and beliefs in your family? Were they values such as respect, hard work, education, and always telling the truth? How were decisions made? What were the views on education and economics? How did religion influence your family's healthcare practices? Now, what happens when your list doesn't match that of your patient or your colleague? Conflict? Misunderstanding? Maybe. We do well not to take it personally, but rather to understand that each person is seeing through his or her cultural filters. The following exercise is an opportunity to discover your cultural values and beliefs.

<u>**Reflective exercise**</u>: **Cultural beliefs and values**
1. *List two beliefs you learned as a child.*
2. *Who did you learn them from?*
3. *Are they still important to you today?*
4. *Have you experienced conflict when your values/beliefs did not match those of another?*
5. *Where do you find common ground with patients and colleagues?*

Were you surprised by your responses? These values and beliefs are unique to "your story." They are what you rely on in times of uncertainty. Julie Lipson (1996), researcher and educator, captures this thought in her definition of culture. For her, it is "the mediator between human beings and chaos, guiding our interactions with each other" (p. 1). As those of us in the field know, healthcare settings can be stressful and may seem chaotic at times, yet our cultural practices help us to manage the situation. Our culture provides the confidence and support.

Next Stop ~ Cultural Awareness

This next step in the journey to cultural competence begins with cultural awareness: an opportunity to acknowledge, appreciate, and accept one's cultural values, beliefs, and unfortunately, biases. These biases, learned as a child and held to be true, can now be re-examined and changed. These "aha" moments of discovery broaden our world view and help us to find common ground with patients and colleagues. Differences, once considered barriers, now give way to bridges of understanding and respect. Think about people and groups that are not part of *your every day*. Are there biases or assumptions you have about them?

Reflective exercise: Cultural Awareness
1. *What ethnic group, religious group, or generational group do you belong to?*
2. *Reflect on some encounter you have had with those who are members of a different group.*
3. *Did you experience any biases or prejudices?*
4. *How did it feel?*

When we encounter people different from ourselves, we have the opportunity to gain an insight into their world. The more opportunities we pursue, the more enlightened we become. Cultural awareness education seminars, field trips, panel discussions, language immersion programs, and case presentations are venues that help to increase cultural awareness. Wade Davis, ethnobiologist, said it well. "The world in which you were born is just one model of reality. Other cultures are not failed attempts at being you: they are unique manifestations of the human spirit." It may seem a little humbling to read this quote, but it does open us to diversity. Cultural humility, the next step on the journey, challenges us to pause, reflect, and be open to another's perspective.

We're getting there ~ the next stop ~ Cultural Humility

What is cultural humility? According to Tervalon and Murray-Garcia, who first coined the phrase, it is "an ongoing process of self reflection and self critique, a way of being aware of our relationship with others and ourselves" (1997 p. 117). It is not static. Cultural humility encourages us not only to recognize and acknowledge our biased assumptions, but to take responsibility for our actions and interactions with others. It calls us to identify power inequities that may exist between us and our patients. Once recognized, how do we deal with the inequity?

Reflective exercise: You are admitting an elderly, limited English speaking woman to your Medical Unit. She is alone. She has few teeth, wears mismatched clothes and smells badly.
1. *What are your immediate thoughts?*
2. *Name one or more biases that spontaneously come to mind.*
3. *Understanding the concept of cultural humility ~ how would your approach her?*

Awareness brings about humility, which brings about further awareness, and ultimately, a change in the way we approach each encounter. Seeing through the eyes of another helps us to discover common ground, enabling us to develop respectful partnerships that are patient centered. We are now ready for the final stage of the journey, cultural competence.

The Final Stage ~ Cultural Competence

Cultural competence is an ongoing process. It begins with an inner desire to know more about other cultures and a willingness to encounter the uncomfortable. Cultural knowledge is acquired with each encounter and every discussion. It summons us to think outside of our "cultural world." Gaining awareness, knowledge, and skill leads to heightened cultural sensitivity and competence. Are you ready?

Reflective exercise: **Cultural competence**
1. *What is motivating me to become culturally competent?*
2. *What do I want/need to know about other cultures . . . and where do I find this information?*
3. *When I experience cultural encounters, how does it feel and what do I learn?*
4. *Whom do I consider a "cultural resource person" in my life?*

Our Journey . . . Putting it into practice

Cultural assessments help to ensure quality care when included with the physical and psychosocial components. In order to provide a cultural assessment, three elements are necessary. First, we must be aware of our cultural beliefs, values, biases, and healthcare practices; second, we must have the knowledge of various ethnic groups; and third, we must have the practical skills necessary to complete a cultural assessment.

In this section we review each of the elements in the author's model, Reflections from Common Ground (Figure 8-1). This model provides you with an opportunity to discover your culture and identify similarities and differences with patients and colleagues. Herein you will find common ground that lays the foundation for providing culturally sensitive and competent care. As you review each element, ask yourself, "How am I the same or different from my patient, and where do I find common ground?"

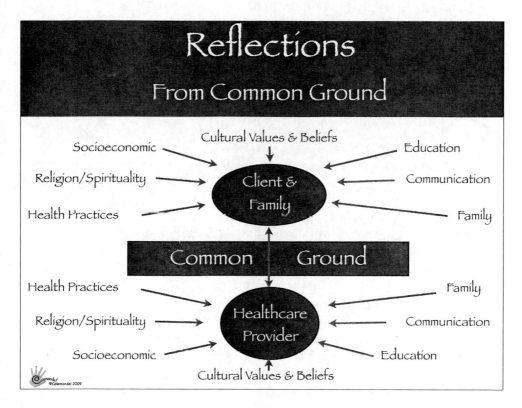

Figure 8-1: Reflections from Common Ground

Our Words . . . Our ways of Communicating

Communication, verbal and nonverbal, is an expression of ourselves – how we reveal ourselves to others. It is our response to encounters with life. Think about your style of communication as you read and reflect on the following:

> **<u>Reflective exercise</u>: Communication**
> 1. *Do I speak loudly or softly?*
> 2. *Do I speak quickly or slowly?*
> 3. *Does the tone of my voice match my words . . . my message?*
> 4. *Does my body language match my words . . . my message?*
> 5. *Do I use facial expressions and gestures to convey my message?*
> 6. *Is eye contact important to my conversation or do I consider it intrusive?*
> 7. *Is touch an acceptable element of my conversation?*
> 8. *Silence – Am I uncomfortable with long periods of silence? Do I use it when I do not want to create conflict or I do not agree with another? It is part of my style?*

Now that you have identified your style of communication, think about your family of origin. Do you see similarities? My guess is that you have heard people comment, "You sound just like your mom . . . your dad . . . your sister . . . brother." Your style is reflective of your lived experience. It's comfortable and fits you perfectly!

The next question is how is my style similar to or different from my patients' and colleagues' style? Do I feel a disconnect when it seems my message is not getting across? We know from "Communication 101" that the more we match the tone, speed, and voice quality of our patient, the more information we share. This reflective technique breaks down barriers and builds rapport. Caution must be taken not to form an opinion about another's unique style of communication; it is just different. A quote by Robert Williams, an educator and researcher, sums it up nicely. He says, "My language is me. It is an extension of my being, my essence. It is a reflection and badge of my culture. Criticism of my language is essentially a direct attack on my self esteem and cultural identity" (Gay 2004 p. 124).

Time . . . How We Use It

Time may be an issue if you are a "to be early is to be on time" person and your patient or colleague is a "get there when I do" person. Time orientation is divided into past, present, and future. While we use all three, two dominate. How we interpret time is culturally learned. In the following exercise, please read all six statements, and then choose two that closely reflect your view of time.

Reflective exercise: My use of time
1. *Respect and honor ancestors*
2. *To be early is to be on time*
3. *I am resistant to change*
4. *The here and now is most important*
5. *Planning for the future is hopeless*
6. *My vacation is planned for next year*

If you are past oriented then respect and honor for the elderly and ancestors in your family/community are important   You seek out their knowledge and wisdom. Resistance to change falls into this category as well. The phrase "can't we go back to way it use to be?" shows a value for past events in contrast with the current situation. It may be difficult to transition into new ways of doing things. Another frequently heard phrase, "Remembering the good old days," offers familiarity and security. Change may cause stress and anxiety. Yet, if given the opportunity to participate in the process of change, you are more likely to accept the outcome.

Present day orientation focuses on today, thus *planning for the future* may seem futile. Besides, the "here and now" feels more comfortable and safe. Your attention to the immediate need of a patient, colleague, or family member may supercede. For you, the "here and now" is important. Attention to the immediate need of patient, colleague, or family member supersedes punctuality. Unfortunately, this may cause others to see you as disorganized in the work setting, but this is not reality. Caring for a patient or taking time to help a colleague helps to ensure that you're meeting their needs.

It you are future oriented, "to be early is to be on time," resonates closely with your thinking. It's all about the future! Vacations are scheduled well in advance. You are motivated to plan for the future by getting a college degree that translates into a better paying job and a secure future. You set timelines to achieve long-term goals. In the workplace you are lauded for your ability to organize your time, set priorities, and get work done on time.

It is essential that we understand that our view of time may be different from others. Working with the patient or colleague to determine the best approach helps to assure understanding and respect for differences.

Reflective exercise: Time
1. *How are you different from your patient population?*
2. *Where do you find common ground?*

My Space – don't come too close!

Spatial orientation is a learned value. From an early age, you were taught, usually tacitly, the appropriate distance between you and family, friends, and outsiders. At home or with extended family, you may be "up close and personal," but this does not translate into acceptable behavior in the public arena. Using what is considered the appropriate space in one situation may not be respectable in another. Have you had the experience of persons invading your "personal space," assuming a familiarity that didn't exist? For them it may just be "who they are." They find it surprising that you are annoyed.

Space, in Western culture, has three dimensions: intimate, personal, and public. Intimate space, designated as zero to eighteen inches, is used by close friends and family. Personal space, eighteen inches to three feet, is used by friends, acquaintances, some colleagues, counselors, and family members. Three to six feet, public space, is used when conducting interviews or business transactions. Other cultural groups may use different parameters. It may be beneficial for you to observe patients' use of space before assuming differently.

Reflective exercise ~ Spatial orientation
1. *When you are talking with friends or family ~ how much distance is between you?*
2. *Does gender or age determine space?*
3. *What do you do when someone "invades" your personal space?*
4. *How are you different from patients or colleagues?*
5. *Where do you find common ground with patients and colleagues?*

Family

The definition of family today may be very different from what it was fifty or even twenty years ago. The U.S. Census Bureau defines family as "people who occupy the same house." Webster's definition relates to descendants from a common progenitor, a tribe, clan, or race. While definitions vary, we do know that families have significant influence in the development of our cultural beliefs, values, behaviors and practices. They provide a social framework that is internalized and accepted as normative and true.

Married with no children, two parent families with children, extended family, single parent, blended, alternative, and same sex partners are all considered, by definition, to be family. Within each of these family structures are assigned and acquired roles and responsibilities. Each designates duty and status. Defined roles provide the support necessary to maintain family harmony during an illness. We know the dynamics of a family can change with the diagnosis of stroke, heart attack, cancer, or diabetes. Who now assumes the role of decision maker and caregiver when a member can no longer fulfill his or her role? What is the response from other members of the family to the change?

Reflective exercise: Family
1. *What was the structure of your family when you were growing up?*
2. *What was your role and responsibility?*
3. *Who was the decision maker?*
4. *What was the role of the sick person?*
5. *What is the structure of your current family? Is it the same or different from that of your family of origin?*
6. *How are you different from your patient population?*
7. *Where do you find common ground?*

Conflict can arise when your cultural view of family responsibilities and roles does not match those of your patients. For example, if you were raised in a two-parent family that espoused an egalitarian view, but your patient comes from a patriarchal family unit with clearly defined gender roles, expectations of behavior may be different. During times of uncertainty for your patient, stress may increase. You can show support and respect by acknowledging difference and working collaboratively with the patient to develop a plan of care that incorporates cultural values and beliefs about family.

Religion/Spirituality

Religion and spirituality may be a source of comfort during difficult times. Religion, thought of as an organized group structure, offers comfort through its set of beliefs and practices based on the teachings of a spiritual icon or leader such as Jesus, Buddha, Mohammed or Brigham Young. The Bible, Qur'an, Book of Mormon, Torah, and other holy texts provide the written word which, when followed, offer a source of well-being and enlightenment. Spirituality is more of an individual approach. It is thought of as a journey in which one seeks awareness and personal meaning from each experience which translates to a better understanding of one's purpose in life. Increased spirituality, as with religion, offers a sense of support and hope when dealing with the unexpected. Both provide a supportive foundation when facing a diagnosis such as terminal cancer of your best friend, a colleague's recent diagnosis of multiple sclerosis, the end stage symptoms of Huntington's chorea in your spouse, or a nephew coping with schizophrenia.

Reflective exercise: Religion/Spirituality
1. *As a child were you part of a religious denomination? . . . Is it the same today?*
2. *Is spirituality an influence in your life?*
3. *In what ways do religion and/or spirituality affect your health? Illness?*
4. *How do your beliefs of religion/spirituality contrast with those of your patients?*
5. *Where do you find common ground?*

There are hundreds of organized churches in the United States and an equal number of spiritual guides, each with beliefs about health and illness, prevention and cure. You cannot possibly know the intricacies of each, but you do have the skill to assess the religious/spiritual needs of the patient. Adherence to religious beliefs and practices for some equates to health and harmony. For others, illness may be seen as a punishment from God or a failure to follow tenets. For one patient this was her reality. She stated assuredly that "God made her bedridden so she would stop what she was doing and listen." The cause of her illness was based on her religious beliefs, and healing would come when she was obedient to God.

Recognizing the importance of religion and spirituality, hospitals across the country have added pastoral care departments. They provide support to patients and families from varied religious affiliations. Together with the patient and pastoral care you can develop a plan of care that acknowledges and incorporates religious and spiritual beliefs.

Education
Education, whether from institutions of learning or life experiences, lays a foundation that influences how we learn. We acquire tools along the way that enable us to take, process, and use new information.

Reflective exercise: Education
1. *How do you learn best? Narrative, Written, Hands On?*
2. *How many years of schooling do you have?*
3. *How does your education and learning style contrast with your patient population?*
4. *Where do you find common ground?*

When you think of your patients, the most important question is "how do you learn best?" rather than "how far did you go in school?" The stigma attached to those who have less than a high school education may prejudice your perspective of the patient's abilities. The patient's ability to read, write, and comprehend information must be assessed. More importantly, though, is the method of learning that is most effective for each person. Your patients may learn by watching videos, engaging in a return demonstration, or participating in group discussions. Or, they may choose to combine all three methods. When you meet the patient and family at their educational level, learning opportunities abound.

Socioeconomic

How your family used money for healthcare in the past may influence how you use it now. Phrases like "we don't go to the doctor unless it is absolutely necessary," or "if I go to the hospital, I'll never come home again," may determine a decision to seek care.

Reflective exercise: Socioeconomic
1. *How would you define your socioeconomic status?*
2. *Does it affect your ability to seek healthcare?*
3. *What would you do if you could not afford to fill a prescription?*
4. *How do your beliefs about money and how it is used contrast with those of your patient population?*
5. *Where do you find common ground?*

The availability of financial resources influences the decision to seek healthcare. In addition, one's socioeconomic status affects how money is managed. From a cultural perspective, money can dictate decisions about healthcare. It is prudent for you to be knowledgeable about available resources for patients and to create an environment that promotes dignity and respect for those whose economic status may be a barrier to care.

Healthcare Practices

Your definition of health and illness determines whether you need to seek professional care or rely on folk practices and proven "home remedies." Professional care, we know, focuses on the biological cause and treatment of an illness, which may include medicine or surgery. At the other end of the spectrum, folk care and home remedies are passed down from one generation to the next. You may have been the recipient of some of these remedies as a child – Vick's® VapoRub® on the chest for a cold, ginger ale and soda crackers for nausea, and carrot syrup for cough. You believed that healing could occur using both approaches.

This belief includes locus of control or your ability or lack of ability to control the situation. It can be either internal or external. An internal locus of control suggests that you have ability to control a situation and to influence the outcome. So, if you follow the plan, eat well, exercise, and get enough sleep, then health is ensured. In contrast, when you subscribe to an external locus of control, efforts and reward are not related. Your health is a result of luck, chance, or faith.

> **Reflective exercise: Cultural healthcare practices**
> 1. *Is your primary approach to healthcare ~ professional? folk? or both?*
> 2. *Do you have an internal or external locus of control?*
> 3. *How do you contrast with your patient population?*
> 4. *Where do you find common ground?*

It is important to note the patient's definition of health and illness and the locus of control when inquiring about cultural health practices and beliefs. This topic will be addressed in greater detail in Chapter 9, *Ancient wisdom . . . Modern Medicine*, as well as in the vignettes.

*   *   *   *

In this chapter we determined that cultural competency is a journey and that it begins with self awareness. The reflective exercises provided you with an opportunity to discover your cultural beliefs, values, biases, and healthcare practices and contrast them with those of patients and colleagues. It is through this process that you find common ground and build the bridge to understanding. Creating an environment that promotes dignity, respect, and openness to other perspectives increases rapport and ensures trusting relationships.

Resources

Andrews, M. M., Boyle, J. S. (2008). *Transcultural concepts in nursing care*. (5th Ed.).New York: Lippincott Williams & Wilkins.

Campinha-Bacote, J. (2003). *The process of cultural competence in the delivery of healthcare services: A culturally competent model of care.* Cincinnati, OH: Transcultural C.A.R.E. Associates.

Gay, G. (2000). *Culturally responsive teaching: Theory, research & practice.* New York: Teachers College Press.

Giger, J. N., Davidhizar, R. E. (2008). Transcultural nursing: Assessment and intervention. (5th Ed.). St Louis, MO: Mosby/Elsevier.

Leininger, M. M. (1991). *Culture care diversity and universality: A theory of nursing.* New York: National League for Nursing Press.

Leininger, M. M., McFarland, M. R. (2002). *Transcultural nursing: Concepts, theories, research and practice.* (3rd Ed.). New York: McGraw-Hill.

Lipson, J. G., Dibble, S. L., Minarik, P. A. (1996). *Culture & Nursing Care: A pocket guide.* San Francisco: UCSF Nursing Press.

McGoldrick, M., Giordano, J., Garcia-Preto, N (2005). *Ethnicity & Family Therapy.* (3rd Ed.). New York: Guilford Press.

Payne, R. (1996). *The Framework of Poverty.* (3rd Ed.). Texas: aha! Process, Inc.

Purnell, L. D., Paulanka, B. J. (2008). Transcultural Health Care: A Culturally Competent Approach. (3rd Ed.). Philadelphia, PA: F. A. Davis Company.

Sandoval, V. A., Adams, S. H. (2001). Subtle skills for building rapport using neuro-linguistic programming in the interview room. *FBI Law Enforcement Bulletin* 1-5.

Spector, R. (2009). *Cultural diversity in health and illness.* (7th Ed.), New Jersey: Pearson/Prentice Hall.

Tervalon, M., Murray-Garcia, J. (1997). Cultural humility versus cultural competence: A criticial, distinction in defining physician training outcomes in multicultural education. *Journal of Health Care for the Poor and Underserved.* (9)2, 117-125.

Ancient Wisdom . . . Modern Medicine

9

Ancient wisdom, folk care, and practices are passed down from one generation to the next. Healing poultices, coining and cupping (use of heat to remove illness from the body), pinching, massage, herbs, and sweat lodges may be used in the curative process. Professional care, on the other hand, refers to modern medicine taught at colleges and universities, and relies on physical exams, blood tests, x-rays, and ultrasounds to diagnose. Pharmaceuticals and surgery provide the cure. Patients may subscribe to both ancient wisdom and modern medicine, depending on circumstances.

Realizing that cultural beliefs and healthcare practices are part of our patient's world view, it may be advantageous to inquire about his or her thoughts as to the cause of the illness. One of my patients presented with upper respiratory symptoms that included congestion and a productive cough for one week. She told me she became ill when she, "opened the window too fast and the wind got insider her." I was taken aback by her unexpected statement and paused while pondering an effective and sensitive response. Additional questions showed an interest on my part to know more, thus she was more open to sharing her concerns.

We, as HCPs, view health, illness, caring, and cure as well-defined concepts within our professional training and education. Our patients, who do not speak our "medical language," may give these concepts different meaning and value. How one perceives and defines health and illness, expectations of behavior and response to treatment is influenced by his or her family of origin.

Reflective exercise: Health and Illness
1. *I know I am healthy when . . .*
2. *I know I am sick when . . .*
3. *The role of the sick person in our family is . . .*
4. *Some of the ways my family shows care when someone is ill . . .*

Responses vary. Our cultural awareness education seminar participants share comments such as, "I know that I am healthy when I wake up and feel well," "I feel happy and energetic," "I don't have pain;" or the opposite, "I have pain," "I'm tired all the time," and "I feel sad." Health or illness can be related to a physical or emotional state or a combination of both.

What was the role of the sick person in your family? Was it his or her job to loll on the couch and have others cater to their every need? Or were they required to "rise above" the discomfort and to continue to function in spite of the illness? It varies according to culture and traditional health beliefs.

Care can be thought of in terms of the verbs: "to care" and "to give care." As HCPs we must acknowledge that the caring practices of various ethnic groups may differ from our prescribed treatment plan, and this may cause misunderstanding and conflict. Knowledge and incorporation of the patient's cultural differences may help bridge the divide we experience with patients.

HEALTH Traditions Model

Cultural Diversity in Health and Illness, by Dr. Rachel Spector (2009), incorporates cultural health traditions and practices of health maintenance, protection, and restoration of health and illness. Heritage consistency, a theory developed by Estes and Zitow, looks at the extent to which one's life is reflective of his or her culture. Dr. Spector expands that concept to acknowledge the importance of traditional health practices and beliefs. Her definition of heritage consistently, "is a means of identification with a traditional ethnocultural heritage leading to the observance of the health/illness beliefs and practices of one's traditional cultural belief system." (2009 p. 9) She sees it as an interwoven influence of one's culture, religion, ethnicity, and socialization. What are the influences of tradition that are necessary to maintain, protect, and restore health? Taking into consideration acculturation, she posits that the more one identifies with traditional culture, the more likely one is to adhere to the cultural values and practices associated with its beliefs of health and illness.

	Physical	Mental	Spiritual
Maintain Health	Proper clothing Proper diet Exercise & Rest	Concentration Social & Family support systems Hobbies	Religious worship Prayer Meditation
Protect Health	Special foods & food combinations Symbolic clothing	Avoid certain people who can cause illness Family activities	Religious customs Superstitions Wearing amulets & other symbolic objects to prevent "Evil Eye" or deter other sources of harm
Restore Health	Homeopathic remedies & liniments Herbal Teas Special foods Massage Acupuncture & Moxibustion	Relaxation Exorcism Curanderos & other traditional healers Nerve teas	Religious rituals – special prayers Meditation Traditional healing Exorcism

Figure 9-1: The nine interrelated facets of HEALTH (physical, mental, and spiritual) and personal methods of maintaining HEALTH , protecting HEALTH, and restoring HEALTH . Used with permission.

Figure 9-1: Traditional HEALTH Model (Personal)
Spector, Rachel E., Cultrual Diversity in Health & Illness, 7th Edition, ©2009, Pgs. 78-79. Reprinted with permission of Pearson Education , Inc. Upper Saddle River, N.J.

Dr. Spector's model, HEALTH Traditions (Figure 9-1: Personal, & Figure 9-2: Communal), focuses on a traditional view of ways to maintain HEALTH, to protect HEALTH, and to restore HEALTH. To differentiate the definition of health from HEALTH, Spector has written it in a small but capitalized format. HEALTH refers to the balance in interrelatedness of one's physical, mental, and spiritual being. The model employs a holistic perspective of the individual or community to discover traditional modes of maintaining, protecting, and restoring health. This information in combination with the HCPs plan of care provides a solid foundation for the continued wellbeing of the patient.

	Physical	**Mental**	**Spiritual**
Maintain Health	Availability of proper shelter, clothing & food Safe air, water & soil	Availability of traditional sources of entertainment, concentration & "rules" of the culture	Availability & promulgation of rules of ritual & religious worship Meditation
Protect Health	Promotion of the knowledge of necessary special foods & food combination, the wearing of symbolic clothing, & avoidance of excessive heat or cold	Provision of the knowledge of what people and situations to avoid, Family activities	The teaching of Religious customs Superstitions Wearing of amulets and other symbolic objects to prevent the "Evil Eye" or how to defray other sources of harm
Restore Health	Resources that provide Homeopathic remedies, liniments, Herbal teas, Special foods, Massage & other ways to restore the body's balance of hot & cold	Traditional healers with the knowledge to use such modalities as: relaxation, exorcism, storytelling, and/or Nerve teas	Availability of healers who use magical and supernatural ways to restore health; including religious rituals, special prayers, meditations, traditional healing &/or exorcism

Figure 9-2: The nine interrelated facets of HEALTH (physical, mental, and spiritual) and communal methods of maintaining HEALTH, protecting HEALTH, and restoring HEALTH. Used with permission.

Figure 9-2: Traditional HEALTH Model (Communal)
pector, Rachel E., Cultrual Diversity in Health & Illness, 7th Edition, ©2009, Pgs. 78-79. Reprinted with permission of Pearson Eduation , Inc. Upper Saddle River, N.J.

What factors does one need to consider to maintain health? For some it may be adequate nutritional intake, exercise, and rest. For others it may mean, in addition to the aforementioned, good relationships with family and friends. For others, it is a strong religious base with rituals that provide well-being. HEALTH maintenance assures that if the patient adheres closely to those practices that promote a healthy lifestyle, then good health is more secure.

HEALTH protection identifies those activities that would protect one from illness or harm. These may include special food, protective objects, or prayers. In some cultural groups such as the Hmong population, people are encouraged to wear red strings about their wrists to protect them from the Dab (an evil spirit that can cause illness), or Chinese American parents may tape a red envelope under the crib of their newborn infant in the neonatal intensive care unit to ensure health.

HEALTH restoration of body, mind, and spirit is achieved through a variety of means and may include home remedies, massage, prayers, religious rituals, and support from family and community. In the Vietnamese culture, coining and cupping may be used to exorcise the illness from the body in order to restore health. Native American populations often use the sweat lodge to provide the restoration of health, physically, and spiritually.

Reflective exercise: As you review the HEALTH Traditions Model . . .
1. *How do you maintain your health?*
2. *Protect your health?*
3. *Restore your health?*
4. *How are your responses different from those of your patient population?*
5. *Where do you find common ground?*

Approaches to Health and Wellness

We cannot be experts on every culture and traditional healing practice. In this section we will focus on three specific approaches, as does Foster in his book Medical Anthropology (1978). These are biomedicine, personalistic, and naturalistic. Each offers a distinct focus on the cause of illness, the treatment plan, cure, and preventative measures that can be used by an individual to ensure wellness.

Biomedicine Approach

Biomedicine, the dominant belief found in the United States and in Western countries, is viewed from the perspective that illness is a result of "cause and effect." Causes include susceptibility to a virus or a bacteria, poor nutrition, exposure to chemicals, injury, or the aging process. Diagnosis is made through the use of laboratory findings, cultures, and x-rays that corroborate physical findings. Treatments include medication, patient education, and follow-up care. Prevention of illness is contingent on the active participation of the individual. Avoidance of pathogens, recreational drugs, alcohol and high risk behavior are on the list. A healthy diet, regular exercise, adequate rest, and vitamin supplements may be other ways a patient maintains health.

As HCPs, this approach is the most familiar to our repertoire, as it is the basis of our educational training: identify the cause, provide a treatment, and cure the illness. Consider our patient with upper respiratory symptoms. With this biomedicine approach, we inquire as to onset and symptoms, take vital signs, perform a physical assessment, and prescribe an antibiotic if the illness is thought to be caused by bacteria, or rest and plenty of fluids if the illness is attributed to a viral infection. Simple and straight-forward.

Personalistic Approach

What if this respiratory illness is caused by something outside of that realm? What if supernatural forces are causing health issues of the body, mind, spirit . . . what then? The personalistic approach, found in the indigenous populations of the Americas as well as Southeast Asia, assumes that the cause of one's illness is secondary to an affliction caused by something paranormal. The "sick person" is the object of punishment by a supernatural being (deity or god), non-human forces (ghost, ancestor, or evil spirit) or by a human being (witch, sorcerer).

Illness may occur because certain rituals of respect were not given to the ancestor. Special days, such as El Dia de Los Muertos in the Mexican tradition or Sweeping the Tomb found in the Chinese and Vietnamese populations, are annual events that give respect to ancestors. On this day, the family goes to the cemetery and cleans the grave of the deceased. They bring this person's favorite food, share stories about the individual, and recognize the importance of that person in their lives. In the pueblo of Pazquero, Mexico, the community rises at midnight and proceeds en masse to the cemetery carrying candles to light the way. They remain at the site throughout the day. This ritual ensures good relationships with the ancestor who is thought to offer protection against illness.

Some cultures believe that non-humans can cause illness as well. In the book, *The Spirit Catches You and You Fall Down*, written by Anne Fadiman (1997), a three-month-old Hmong child becomes ill after her sister slams the door. The parents believed that her soul had left her body and become lost. The emergency room physician ordered an x-ray and told the parents the child had a "bronchipneumonia or tracheobronchitis." He ordered antibiotics – a biomedicine approach. Following the emergency room visit, the family sought out the clan's txiv neb, a Hmong healer. They requested a ceremony that would return the child's soul and thus restore health.

In addition to rituals and healing ceremonies, cures may include offering prayers, lighting candles to lift spells, and visits by clergy. You may also see patients wearing amulets or carrying other protective objects that are thought to ensure health. As HCPs, we need to ask the patient what is needed to restore health. Prevention in the personalistic approach includes maintaining good relationships not only with the living, but also with ancestors and deities.

Naturalistic Approach

Health returns when balance is restored in the Naturalistic approach. It is all about balance! This approach to health and illness is found primarily in Asian countries, Latin America, and in the Philippines. The cause of an illness is an exposure to excessive hot or cold, creating an imbalance that leads to illness. Whether an illness is deemed hot or cold is based on the health beliefs and practices of the individual or group.

Treatment comes in the form of balancing a hot condition with a cold solution, and vice versa. It may be helpful to ask about what the patient believes is needed to restore balance. If a hospitalized patient is refusing certain foods or medicines, that may be our cue to inquire if other foods (deemed hot or cold) would be appreciated. Prevention is assured with one's ability to maintain the balance of mind, body, and spirit. Eating the right foods, getting enough rest, and avoiding disagreements with family and friends may indeed ensure a more healthy life.

These three approaches – biomedicine, personalistic, and naturalistic – may coexist with one another. While in Western countries, biomedicine is dominant, other treatment modalities may also be applied. We may not be aware of it; we need to ask.

Locus of control is an important variable that must be understood in order to plan care that is effective and consistent with the patient's beliefs and practices. People with an internal locus of control believe in their ability to control the environment, thus protecting their health. The belief in adherence to a healthy lifestyle, which includes annual physical exams, good nutritional intake, and daily exercise, ensures a healthy life.

Those with an external locus of control believe that they do not have the power or ability to effect maintenance of health. Fate, luck, chance, and God are the controllers. This sometimes is referred to as a "fatalistic" approach – always thinking the worst. As a HCP, you may hear some one say, "if it is God's will," thus and such will happen, implying that health maintenance is out of his or her control. The patient may not be interested in wellness programs, stop smoking programs, or exercise regimes that are suggested. As HCPs, we can acknowledge the patient's belief, and share some internal locus of control methods that may enable the patient to see positive outcomes and renewed sense of well-being.

> **Reflective exercise**: **My approach to health is usually . . .**
> 1. *My approach to health is usually Biomedicine . . . Personalistic . . . Naturalistic?*
> 2. *My patient population is usually . . . ?*
> 3. *My locus of control is internal or external?*
> 4. *My patient population's locus of control?*

It's All About Balance ~
Four Humors . . . Hot/Cold . . . Yin/Yang . . . Wind

Four Humors ~ Hot & Cold

How does one restore balance or, better yet, maintain balance? The Four Humors, (Figure 9-3), date back to the beginning of the second century when Hippocrates, a Greek physician, first coined the term. These four elements, considered ether-like qualities emanating from the brain, balance the body to prevent illness from entering. This theory of disease existed even into the 19th century.

Element	Body	Temperature	Moisture	Personality	Season
Air	**Blood**	Hot	Wet	Sanguine	Spring
Fire	**Yellow Bile**	*Hot*	*Dry*	*Choleric*	*Summer*
Water	**Phlegm**	Cold	Phlegmatic	Wet	Winter
Earth	**Black Bile**	Cold	Dry	Melancholic	Autumn

Figure 9-3: Four Body Humors & Complimental Elements

102

Listed are the components of the Four Body Humors – blood, yellow bile, phlegm, and black bile, including element, temperature, moisture, personality, and season. If one looks closely it is easy to see the interrelatedness of the categories. For example, phlegm is associated with cold, wet, and winter, a season when upper respiratory symptoms usually occur. Look again. Do you see any other "related" categories?

A lighter note referencing the humors was given by our tour guide in Annapolis, MD, *Squire Douglas*, who shared with us the four main ways to rebalance and restore health in the 18th and 19th century.

1. Since the **mouth** was the main entrance of the outside world into the body, an emetic was given to clean out the stomach.
2. If you think the **stomach** was bad, you can imagine what is in the lower bowel. Therefore, they gave cathartics.
3. Since **blood** carries disease through the body, leeches and the scalpel were used to drain out the infirmities.
4. Lastly, **blistering** was used to drain infection out of the body. Redness and drainage caused by blistering the skin was evidence of the illness leaving the body. A hot coin was used.

Yin & Yang Theory

The above symbol, Yin (black) and Yang (white), represents the ancient Chinese understanding of the foundation of the universe. It is thought that the energies of Yin and Yang make everything happen. One element cannot exist without the other; they are complementary. Similar to the hot and cold theory, Yin and Yang strives to balance contrasting elements. The Yin and Yang chart (Figure 9-4) shows the contrasts between them. If Yang, the masculine force is overwhelming, then there is excessive heat which injures the spirit. Severe pain follows. Excessive cold, the feminine Yin factor, causes injury to the body creating swelling. Therefore, the onset of pain followed by swelling indicates a disharmony in the spirit has injured the body. But if swelling comes first, followed by pain then a disharmony in the body has harmed the spirit. Cure comes in the form of balance, mediating excessive heat or cold through the use of remedies such as herbal therapy, acupuncture, coining, or cupping.

YIN	YANG
Female	Male
Cold	Hot
Darker	Lighter
Found inside body	Found on surface of body
Corresponds to night	Corresponds to day
Stands for confusion & turmoil	Stands for peace & harmony
Stands for conservation	Stands for destruction
Created earth	Created heaven

Figure 9-4: Yin and Yang Chart

In the case of the patient with an upper respiratory infection, symptoms may include cough, fatigue, and yellow sputum. A traditional healer may diagnose heat clogging in the lungs and prescribe acupuncture, herbal tea, and rest in order to restore balance of Yin and Yang.

Wind Theory

Once wind gets inside you, illness will occur. One day a Mexican American father brought his five-year-old daughter to the clinic. She had painful and frequent urination. From my biomedicine perspective and experience, I considered a urinary tract infection, vesicoureteral reflux, and possible sexual abuse, as urinary tract infection symptoms are uncommon in children under the age of five. She looked well. I asked the father, "what do you think made her sick?" He responded, "when I took her outside the wind got inside of her."

The idea that wind, considered a menacing element, causes illness is a cultural health belief found in the Hmong, Cambodian, and Vietnamese cultures as well as Mexican. Symptoms congruent with the wind are fatigue, feeling of hot or cold, headache, restlessness, and decreased energy level. While these complaints could represent a variety of conditions, cure may come in the form of moxibustion (heat). It is a belief that heat has a therapeutic and balancing effect on the body, and through this process wind is released and health restored.

Cures and other remedies

Coining is a heat treatment method frequently used to restore balance to the body. After an ointment is applied, a heated coin is placed on the affected site. The coin is pressed firmly against the skin and drawn down in one direction, hopefully without breaking the skin. This is repeated several times. If a dark blood appears under the skin, it is assumed that the treatment is working. If the site is only mildly red, the patient may need further treatments. On physical exam, the HCP would see ecchymotic stripes in symmetrical rows. This would confirm that the patient did have "bad wind!"

Cupping, a similar method, is used when there is excessive Yin, as seen with sore muscles and body aches. A small heated cup-like form is applied to the skin, which causes a vacuum like suction to occur as it cools, thus rendering the noxious element ineffective and released from the body. Each application of a cup may take fifteen to twenty minutes. Again, on physical examination the HCP will see symmetrical, vertical rows of circular, non-raised, ecchymotic marks. It is thought that the greater the bruise, the greater the illness. This treatment removes cold elements and increases circulation.

Following the treatment, the patient is admonished to avoid taking a bath or drinking cold water because when water gets inside the body, it may block the wind from getting out, thus making symptoms worse. In talking with patients who hold a strong belief in this process, many will say they actually feel better after the treatment.

Restoring health may also come in the form of pinching. This procedure is especially effective with headaches, fatigue, loss of appetite, visual changes and to release wind from the body. For a headache, the procedure begins with rubbing a mentholated balm into the area, then placing the fingers and thumbs on both temples, slowing moving them in a massage-like fashion across the forehead toward a spot between the eyes. The area between the eyes is then pinched and twisted. As with coining and cupping, if petechiae or ecchymosis occurs the treatment is deemed successful. It may be used on other areas of the body as well.

Massage provides yet another avenue to release the wind. Balm or lotion is rubbed onto the body to increase the blood flow and to relax the muscles and the mind. Following the massage, the skin may be pinched and lifted to facilitate the release of the wind.

Other forms of Treatment

Acupuncture

The National Institute of Health has reviewed and scientifically analyzed several studies advocating the effectiveness of acupuncture. In 1997, a panel identified conditions that they felt would benefit from this adjunct therapy including addiction, stroke, rehabilitation, headache, carpal tunnel, and asthma (National Institute of Health, 1997). In addition the World Health Organization lists several conditions in which acupuncture is an effective treatment. These include upper respiratory infections, gastrointestinal issues, gynecological problems, and muscular disorders.

Acupuncture, a treatment based on Chinese medicine, has been around for thousands of years, but is just now recognized for its healing properties and only recently funded by some insurance companies. Considered a cold treatment to remove excessive Yang, it restores balance. The practice of puncturing the body to cure disease or relieve pain is done with a variety of needles, each having a specific purpose. Within the body, Chinese tradition asserts there is a vital life force called *Qi*. When the *Qi* is depleted or imbalanced, physical, emotional, or mental illness can ensue. Meridians, the acupuncture sites for needle insertion, are thought to be the pathways where our *Qi* flows. Needle insertion rebalances this flow.

Sweat Lodge

On a visit to the Paiute Shosone Indian Cultural Center in Bishop, California, our tour guide, a young Paiute Indian, shared information about his history and the cultural beliefs of his people. We discussed the sweat lodge and its healing properties. He must have gotten the sense that I needed healing because he offered to set up a time for a sweat lodge experience! I was surprised by his openness and generosity to someone not of native ancestry.

The Native American cultural belief of harmony and oneness with nature is revealed in the spiritual renewal and purification ceremony held in sweat lodges. Four recognized elements, fire, water, earth, and air, are similar to those found in the Four Humors. These ceremonies, considered sacred events, can be used to heal an illness, to prepare for another ceremony or to seek guidance. Sage and sweet grass, both considered to have healing properties, are used along with cedar. Rocks are heated prior to the ceremony and placed in strategic locations. The doors are closed and prayers begin with a welcome for the spirits to join the participants.

Reiki

As HCPs we cannot know every possible nontraditional treatment, but I am always amazed when I hear about a new form, even though it has been around for hundreds of years. At a recent seminar I was presenting, a participant shared information about Reiki and now I'd like to share it with you. Reiki was developed by Dr. Mikao in the 1880s in response to his student's inquiries about the healing abilities of Jesus and other spiritual healers. Reiki comes from two Japanese words: *rei*, which means "God's wisdom or higher power"; and *ki*, which is life force energy. It is the restorative nature that provides stress reduction and promotes healing. Placing one's hand just above the body and using various hand positions transfers the energy from the practitioner to the patient. Treating the whole person in this manner brings about feelings of peace, harmony, and wellbeing.

Laughter Club

Laughter is the best medicine. The laughter club, first conceived by Dr. Madan Katana, a Bombay physician, takes advantage of the therapeutic value and contagious nature of laughing to promote wellness. There are over 400 clubs around the world and 72% of the members report improved interpersonal relationship with coworkers, 85% say it has improved their self confidence and 66% suggest that it has improved their ability to concentrate. We all need a little laughter every day!

Herbal Therapy

The decision when to pick, where to pick, and how to prepare plants all determine the effectiveness of herbal therapy. At a recent Transcultural Nursing conference, I spent time with a Native Hawaiian registered nurse who was also a healer. As a child she had been chosen by her grandfather to become the next healer in their community. She shared stories of leaving the house at midnight during a full moon in order to pick the herbs needed for her grandfather's patients. The tradition was passed from grandfather to granddaughter. Although she wants to write all this information down for the next generation, she has already met with resistance from her community as it is not in keeping with their oral tradition.

Herbs, like acupuncture, have become a part of mainstream medicine. While effective, they are not without possible side effects, thus discussion regarding their properties with patients is essential. There are a multitude of herbs that have medicinal properties, and it is best to inquire if your patient is using them on a regular basis and for what purpose. Some of the commonly uses herbs are sage, chamomile, and ginseng.

Sage, used aromatically in the sweat lodge, is thought to purify and cleanse the body, mind, and spirit. It may also be used for sleep, sore throat, breath cleansing and fever. It has been known to be used as a sage tea rubdown or bath as well as to drink or chew to cleanse the body's system of impurities. Chamomile, used by many as a means of relaxation, is thought to have a sedative and quieting effect, especially after a hectic day at work. Combined with a warm bath, it may be helpful to relax muscles. Ginseng, a very popular herb, is thought to promote and improve male fertility as well as to enhance the immune system. For backpackers planning a trek at high elevations, it is said that by taking it three days prior to a trip and then the first two days on the trail, one can avoid altitude sickness. Since dehydration aggravates altitude sickness, it is vital to drink plenty of water at high elevations, whether ginseng is used or not.

It is always best for the HCP to inquire about the herbs and over-the-counter treatments currently used by the patient and to discuss potential side effects and possible interactions with their current medications.

Reflective exercise: **Healing treatments**
1. *What home remedies did your family use?*
2. *Were they helpful?*
3. *Do you still use them today?*
4. *Besides the healing treatments we discussed, what other healing modalities do your patients subscribe to in times of illness?*
5. *Are they incorporated into the plan of care?*

Healers

Healers have been a part of cultures for thousands of years. A Native American man shared at the Pomo Indian Conference that the elders of his tribe had selected him to be a healer. The young man was surprised by this, but then spent time in contemplation before responding to the request. In some cultures one may be "called" by the divine to serve as healer, or identified by parents who deem their child ready to follow in their footsteps. This was the case of the Native Hawaiian registered nurse, whose grandfather selected her. Much of the information, beliefs, and practices pass down from one generation to another orally. These cultural beliefs and healthcare practices are considered believable and efficacious. Practices may include herbal therapy, massage, and a spiritual component as well, using prayers or lighting candles. Here is a list of healers from different cultural groups. Can you match them up?

Reflective exercise: Match the correct healer with their culture

1. Curandero .... A. Korean
2. Folk Healer .... B. Roma
3. Hanui .... C. Mexican
4. Hilot .... D. Hmong
5. Txiv Neb .... E. Euro American
6. Drabarni .... F. African American
7. Medicine man/woman .... G. Filipino
8. Physican/Nurse Practitioner .... H. Native American

Answers: 1-C; 2-F; 3-A; 4-G; 5-D; 6-B; 7-H; 8-E

*   *   *   *

Ancient wisdom, folk care practices, and healers are still an integral part of the lives of the patients we care for on a daily basis. Modern medicine is thought to have healing powers as well. The combination of the two modalities for some patients is the key to recovery from illness. An inquisitive HCP seeks out information from the patient to assure that all possibilities have been uncovered. Together they develop a plan of care that incorporates cultural beliefs, values, and health practices into the healing process.

Resources

Amerson, R. (2008). Reflections on a conversation with acurandera. *Journal of Transcultural Nursing.* (19)4, 384-387.

Andrews, M. M., Boyle, J. S. (2008). *Transcultural concepts in nursing care.* (5th Ed.).New York: Lippincott Williams & Wilkins.

Campinha-Bacote, J. (2003). The process of cultural competence in the delivery of healthcare services: A culturally competent model of care. Cincinnati, OH: Transcultural C.A.R.E. Associates.

Fadiman, A. (1997). *The Spirit Catches You and You Fall Down.* New York: Farrar, Straus and Giroux.

Foster, G. M. (1978). *Medical Anthropology.* New York: John Wiley and Sons.

Galanti, G. A. (2004). *Caring for patients from different cultures.* (4th Ed.). Philadelphia: University of Pennsylvania Press.

Giger, J. N., Davidhizar, R. E. (2008). *Transcultural nursing: Assessment and intervention.* (5th Ed.). St Louis, MO: Mosby/Elsevier.

Helsel, D., Mochel, M., Bauer, R. (2005). Chronic Illness and Hmong Shamans. *Journal of Transcultural Nursing.* (16)1, 150-154.

Hodge, F. S., Pasqua, B. A. Marquez, C. A., Cantrell, B. G. (2001). Utilizing storytelling to promote wellness in American Indian communities. *Journal of Transcultural Nursing.* 13(1), 6-11.

Jackson, L. E. (1993). Understanding, eliciting, and genotiating clients' multicultural health beliefs. *Nurse Practitioner.* 18(4), 30-42.

Jones, P. S., Zhang, X. E., Siegl, K. J., Melies, A. (2002). Caregiving between two cultures: An integrative experience. *Journal of Transcultural Nursing.* (13)3, 210-217.

Leininger, M. M. (1991). *Culture care diversity and universality: A theory of nursing.* New York: National League for Nursing Press.

Leininger, M. M., McFarland, M. R. (2002). *Transcultural nursing: Concepts, theories, research and practice.* (3rd Ed.). New York: McGraw-Hill.

Lipson, J.G., Dibble, S.L. (2005). Culture & Clinical Care. (8th Ed.). San Francisco, CA: UCSF Nursing Press

Marchione, M. (2009). Alternative medicine goes mainstream. *Napa Valley Register.* June 8, 2009. p. C5.

McGoldrick, M, Giordano, J., Garcia-Preto, N. (2005). *Ethnicity & Family Therapy.* (3rd Ed.). New York: Guilford Press

Purnell, L. D., Paulanka, B. J. (2008). Transcultural Health Care: A Culturally Competent Approach. (3rd Ed.). Philadelphia, PA: F. A. Davis Company.

Sandoval, V. A., Adams, S. H. (2001). Subtle skills for building rapport using neuro-linguistic programming in the interview room. *FBI Law Enforcement Bulletin* 1-5.

Siatkowshi, A. A. (2007). Hispanic acculturation: A concept analysis. *Journal of Transcultural Nursing.* (18)4, 316-323.

Spector, R. (2009). *Cultural diversity in health and illness.* (7th Ed.), New Jersey: Pearson/Prentice Hall.

Thompson, S. B., Chien, E. (2006). Chinese medicine gaining respectibility in west. *San Francisco Chronicle.* June 27, 2006.

Vigil, D. (2006). Thousands at cemetery for tomb sweeping rites. *San Francisco Chronicle.* April 3, 2006.

Vivian, C., Dundes, L. (2004). The crossroads of culture and health among the Roma (Gypsies). *Journal of Nursing Scholarship.* (38)1, 86-91.

Yin and Yang. Retrieved October 2006 from the World Wide Web. Acupunture.com.au - Yin and Yang

The Pressure To Choose . . .
My Grandmother Or My Nurse Midwife
(Mexican)

10

Lucia - burped, bringing a tinge of rosiness to her plump cheeks. What a thing to do when the midwife's here!

And Mary, her midwife, was going on again about Lucia's weight too, when the whole Ramos family – well, all of the women anyway – had been so clear that she needed to eat more. Even a month or two ago when she seemed to spend more time in the baño sick to her stomach, her mother Rosa and her abuelita were bringing her chicken soup and tortillas as soon as she came out of the door. The soup was the kind she liked, with a thin layer of fat floating on top and big chunks of chicken. And of course her grandmother had made the tortillas herself. How could she refuse?

"So Lucia. What did you have for breakfast?"

"It wasn't much, Mary," Lucia murmured softly, as she looked down at the buttons straining on her green blouse. Lucia had never been lacking as far as her senos like some of those skinny girls. They were even bigger now that she was expecting, and Luis, her novio, loved them that way. He loved her shiny black hair too, especially when she wore it down and not tied, but he was really delighted with her full figure.

"Yes?" Mary pressed.

"Only a little egg and some pan dulce and chorizos," whispered Lucia. And hot chocolate, she remembered, but decided not to mention. She liked Mary, but was afraid of her, a woman with a job that was so important; lots of education.

"Well, you're still gaining too much, Honey. I've been in this business too long not to know better than you what's good for you. You're only four month along, and have gained almost what you should by the time of delivery! Have you been cutting back on the rice and tortillas? I can't be there to make sure you eat properly, but your blood sugar is way too high. Do you understand, Lucia? In a month you won't even be able to get out of bed. And the birth will be dangerous for you and the baby if your keep gaining like this. You're just on the brink of diabetes, you know."

Lucia's mind wandered as Mary droned on; she suddenly felt cold, fear gripping her as salient words like "dangerous" and "diabetes" poked through the verbal haze. She'd heard this all before, of course. Her mind searched for a response, so that she could be in her favor again.

"Cuaresma, that's that time before Jesus came back – how you call it? – that's coming up, Mary and we're supposed to eat less then. Maybe I can give up some food I like too much."

Even as she said it, Lucia knew that her mother and especially her abuelita would say that she shouldn't cut back at all; they'd suggest that she just be extra sweet and take lots of naps and eat for the baby instead. Pregnant women deserved special privileges even during Lent. They'd almost convinced Padre Humberto on that point.

And hadn't they both had babies? They know what's good for me, don't they? Why is Mary always telling me the opposite from what they say? I've never asked, Lucia thought, but I bet Mary's never even HAD a baby.

Cultural Beliefs & Values

Our scenario highlights those highly held values in the Mexican culture: respect and compliance with the elderly and those in authority. We can easily see Lucia's dilemma – who to listen to about her diet. This poses a difficulty for Mary, her midwife, as well, because she knows that the outcome of doing nothing to address the dietary habits of Lucia may have a "dangerous" effect on both mother and child. She admonishes Lucia at each visit to watch what she eats. Care in the Mexican culture is shown by family support; physical, emotional, and financial. The mother and grandmother show care by encouraging Lucia to rest and "eat for two." The findings of an ethnostudy of Mexican-American culture (Staisak 1991) highlight that care means "everything or almost everything," which translates into being with family and bienestar (wellbeing). During pregnancy, women are encouraged to rest, eat well, and avoid stress. These cultural health practices influence decisions and actions. Listed below are other cultural beliefs and values found in the Mexican culture.

Mexcian Cultural Beliefs & Values

- Respect for the elderly and those in authority
- Family loyalty and support
- Interdependence within extended family
- Fatalistic
- Benefits of folk care and healing practices
- Here and now

We as HCPs face similar situations when the cultural beliefs and values of our patients differ from our view of care. The goal is to find some common ground. Encouraging patients to participate actively in their own care may be the first step. What are their opinions about the care received? By acknowledging the importance and value of this information we establish rapport. As noted, family is everything in Lucia's world view. It may be helpful to invite the mother and grandmother to the next clinic visit.

Reflective exercise: Cultural Beliefs, Values, and Health Practices

1. *How do your cultural beliefs and values compare and contrast with Lucia's?*
2. *Have you had similar experiences with patients?*
3. *What did you do? Did it work?*
4. *Now that you have this information ~ how would you approach care differently?*

Familia . . . Familism . . . Family is Everything

Family first. The term *familism* extends the value of family to include others such as abuelos (grandparents), compadres (god parents), sobrinos (niece/nephew), and primos, (cousins) y mas (more). This extended family shares responsibility to nurture and care for children, to provide financial support, to assist with healthcare needs, and to provide a listening ear. It can be thought of as an interdependent system in which help is readily available in any situation. There is a strong sense of loyalty and support for one another.

In the traditional Mexican family, the father is the head of the household. The term *machismo* is often used to describe his role as provider, protector, and decision-maker. This role is taken very seriously. Recently a Mexican-American man, a vineyard worker, presented to the clinic with complaints of back pain which had been going on for several days. This particular day in February was cold, wet, and dreary. I certainly felt his discomfort and admired him for his endurance. Realizing his temperature was 102 degrees, I listened to heart and lungs. This was not a lumbar strain as he thought: it was pneumonia. After providing him with antibiotics and counseling him to go home immediately, I was informed that he "still had work to do" and would leave at the end of the day. Doing his job and providing for family were more important than his own health.

The role of the mother is caregiver and nurturer. She provides stability to the family. Mothers are highly esteemed and hold great influence over their children throughout their lifetime. As a result of economic pressures in the U. S., more women are seeking employment outside of the home, thus adding more responsibilities to their days. It is not uncommon for the HCP to hear a Mexican-American woman tell of a variety of somatic complaints that result from long hours both at home and at work. One of my patients shared how she rose at 5:30 a.m., fixed her husband's breakfast, prepared her children for school, and then went to work. At 4:00 p.m. she picked up her children at school, grocery shopped, prepared dinner, and then went to bed at 11:00 p.m., only to repeat this pattern the next day. Though she was tired, she took her role as caregiver and nurturer more seriously than her exhaustion.

Children within the Mexican community are valued and cared for in a very protective environment. At an early age they are taught the values of *familism* and *respeto*. They may have responsibilities such as childcare for the younger siblings and other household chores, which is in keeping with the value placed on family support. They are expected to do well in school and to bring pride to the family.

The elderly, held in high regard, are also thought wise and knowledgeable. In our scenario, Lucia's grandmother encourages her to "eat for two." Unfortunately, this is in direct conflict with Mary's advice to cut down her caloric intake. Lucia is caught in the middle. She neither wants to disrespect her HCP nor her grandmother. How can the HCP resolve this situation? Taking the cultural value of respect for the elderly into consideration, one possible solution may be to include the grandmother in the planning process. This acknowledges her status and shows an interest in her perspective.

Reflection exercise: Family
1. *How have you heard "machismo" defined?*
2. *What positive and negative terms are used to describe this term?*
3. *How is your family similar to or different from the one described?*
4. *In what ways do you promote family involvement?*

Communication . . . Verbal and Non-Verbal

Spanish is the primary language spoken in 62% of the Mexican households in the United States (U.S. Census 2007). Time spent in this country does not always equate to English proficiency. A Mexican-American patient of mine has lived here for thirty years and does not speak English well but uses a combination of English and Spanish. When asked why she has never learned English, her response surprised me. She indicated that once her husband retired from vineyard work, they planned to return to Mexico. She said that both her husband and son spoke English and, therefore, she saw no need to learn the language.

Both verbal and nonverbal communication are bound by *respeto* (respect). Use of the formal *usted* instead of the informal *tu* when speaking Spanish to an elderly person shows respect. When conversing with children, on the other hand, *tu* is appropriate. Standing when the HCP enters the room shows respect for the position. A handshake is acceptable at that time as well.

The communication style of the Mexican patient varies, depending on the situation. With family and friends, in a social venue, the conversation may seem loud, fast, and expressive. In a clinical setting, voice quality is quieter and eye contact is usually minimal. If the HCP speaks Spanish, one can expect a more expressive and louder conversation along with the use of hand gestures. Emphasis on certain words, gestures, and facial expressions reflects the importance of a situation. During a conversation when Spanish is spoken, it may seem that one word flows directly into the next. According to Zoucha (2004, p.266), this is called apocopation. It is a style of communication used when the end of one word is a vowel, as is the beginning of the next word in a phrase. For example the phrase "¿Como esta usted?" may sound like "¿comoustausted?" It is at this time in the dialogue that the HCP may request "un poco mas despacio, por favor" . . . a little slower please. When patients understand that you really do want to know what is being said, they are more than willing to slow down.

Starting the conversation with small talk before engaging in the discussion of the appointment is an important way to establish rapport with the patient. It is referred to as "setting the stage," or the preamble before the interviewing process begins. You can start by asking how the family is doing and about life in general before discussing the purpose for the appointment. Showing an interest in the patient's life helps establish a respectful relationship

Respeto/Simpatico
Personalismo refers to a personal relationship that promotes harmony and respect. Once established, it leads to a more interactive dialogue with the Mexican patient. *Simpatico* (smooth relationship) encourages a conversation that is respectful and avoids conflict or disagreement. Expressions of anger within and outside of the family generally are discouraged. Assertiveness that displays a differing opinion or a demand for clarification may be seen as rude or insensitive to others' feelings. In this context, it is vital for HCPs to know that an expression of agreement may not always mean agreement, but could have been offered to avoid conflict and promote harmony. The key here is to watch the body language. Does it match the message?

Communication Strategies
- Speak slowly and clearly if limited English is spoken
- Do not raise your voice
- Use minimal eye contact
- Promote personalismo y simpatico y respeto
- How does each of those qualities match your style of communication?
- What do you need to consider changing?

Here and Now . . . Carpe diem
Past and present day orientations are dominant in the Mexican-American culture. Past orientation is shown in annual events such as *El Dia de los Muertos*, The Day of the Dead, which celebrates those who have died. Ancestors are thought to still be part of the family even in death. They guide and protect those who are alive. Recognition on this special day includes preparation of the deceased's favorite food, cleaning the grave site, and telling stories about those who have gone before. It is a way of showing respect and appreciation for their lives.

The value of "here and now" refers to the importance of the moment. Present day orientation values attentiveness to the current situation. In the movie "*La Familia*," the eldest son comments on the amount of money his father spent on his sister's wedding: "It took him years to repay, but what's money for?" The belief is that there is no guarantee for future plans; consequently, do what must be done today. In my practice, some of my Mexican patients arrive early for the appointment, some late, and others on time. The reasons vary. It may relate to the lack of transportation or the need of another family member. It is never intentional. Patients always offer an apology and show a genuine appreciation for the flexibility shown by the HCP.

The future, however, is still held in high regard, especially in relation to the children and education. With each succeeding generation, acculturation to American ways leads to a more future-oriented frame of reference, which may cause a conflict with parents and elders.

Health Beliefs

There are many beliefs about health and illness in the Mexican tradition. "Good health to many Mexican Americans is to be free of pain, able to work, and spend time with the family. In addition, good health is a gift from God and from living a good life." (Zoucha 1998) Illness due to wind getting inside the body or to an imbalance of hot and cold (humoral theory) was introduced to the indigenous population of Mexico in the 16th century by the Spaniards. Over time it blended with the herbal medicines and folk beliefs of the native people. Illness, in addition to an imbalance in hot and cold, can also come about as a result of stress, tension in personal relationships, or one's relationship with the Supreme Being.

God may also determine whether one is to recover from an illness. The fatalistic view subscribed to by the Mexican patient implies that health or illness is out of his control. Any effort on the individual's part does not affect the outcome, positive or negative. It is "God's will." Unfortunately, this belief in an external locus of control may negate the patient's acceptance of responsibility, thus limiting participation in the plan of care.

Healers, known as *curanderos* in the Mexican culture, espouse a holistic approach to health and illness. They receive this gift through "a calling," an apprenticeship, or an innate ability to diagnose and cure. Healing comes through the use of folk practices such as massage, herbs, prayers, lighted candles, and intercession with the divine on behalf of the patients. At a recent healthcare conference three local curanderas spoke. The moderator shared the healers' concern of "coming out into the open." How would they be viewed by western health professionals? However, the response from our group was overwhelmingly positive. It opened doors for future dialogue about current use of folk medicine as well.

Reflective exercise: Health and healers . . .
1. *How do you collaborate with patients who have a "fatalistic" approach ~ an external locus of control?*
2. *Who are the healers in your area?*
3. *What more would you like to know about them and what they do?*
4. *How would you incorporate these practices into your plan of care?*

Childbearing Practices

Prenatal Care

Motherhood is held in high regard in the Mexican-American community. The cultural values of the importance of family and spiritual beliefs, such as the holiness of the Virgin de Guadalupe (protector during pregnancy), are a source of support for pregnant women. They are discouraged from heavy lifting, bending, extended standing, or heavy work. The husband, seen as protector and economic provider, tries to decrease the stress from the outside world. Female family members, especially the grandmother as in Lucia's case, encourage her to participate in traditional beliefs and practices that ensure a healthy baby. It is common for the grandmother to live with the family during the last few weeks or months of the pregnancy and through the *cuarentena*, the period of 40 days following the birth.

Pregnancy is not considered an illness and, therefore, early prenatal care is not thought to be necessary. Barriers such as language, availability of transportation, and economics may also affect the mother's decision not to seek early prenatal care. It is interesting to note that acculturation may or may not play a significant role in deciding to take a more traditional approach to the childbearing experience. A research paper called "*The Mother Study*," done in Watsonville, California, found that regardless of the level of acculturation to the U.S. culture, pregnant Mexican-American women returned to more traditional pregnancy beliefs and practices espoused by female kin and especially their grandmothers. Traditional cultural practices that are beneficial include the following suggestions: eating right (come bien), walking (camina), and don't worry (no se preocupe). (LaGuná 2003)

Reflective exercise: During the prenatal period
1. *Do you encourage participation of female members of the family, especially the grandmother?*
2. *Are spouses part of decision-making process?*
3. *In what ways are the patient's cultural values, beliefs, and practices supported during the prenatal period?*
4. *Is there bilingual/bicultural professional staff available?*
5. *Does the educational material (brochures and classes) reflect the language and educational level of the patient?*

Intrapartum

Lucia, similar to other Mexican women, may come to the hospital late in labor because of concerns about medical intervention. Once there, family members help to decrease her stress. Traditionally, women are attended by the female members of her family, her sisters, aunts, mother, and grandmother. The father may remain in the waiting room or continue to work. While this may appear to the HCP as disinterest, culturally it is considered appropriate behavior. This practice is changing as fathers are taking a more active role in attendance at prenatal and La Maze classes. Extended family may occupy the waiting room. It may be helpful to discuss visitor policies with Lucia during a prenatal appointment. Understanding the importance of *familiso*, staff can work with her to accommodate family. Demonstrating cultural knowledge assures the mother that her needs and those of the family are known and respected.

Cultural beliefs during pregnancy include adherence to the "hot and cold" theory. Pregnancy is considered a "hot" condition. Cold, in the form of air, food, or medication is avoided. When are those times during the labor period in which Lucia may be exposed to the cold, thus losing heat? Every time the sheets are pulled back, a vaginal examination is performed, or ice chips are placed at the bedside table. Walking, an important cultural value during labor, is encouraged. Inactivity is thought to result in the loss of amniotic fluid, which may cause the fetus to stick (se pega) to the uterus. Performing a cultural assessment during the prenatal phase provides hospital staff information that assists them in caring for the woman.

Reflective exercise: Expectations during the intrapartum phase
1. *How are visitors accommodated during this time?*
2. *Do you notice the patient avoiding cold beverages or ice chips?*
3. *In what ways do you welcome family members to participate in care?*
4. *Is there bilingual/bicultural professional staff available to translate?*

Postpartum . . . Loss of Heat

Defending against the heat loss of childbirth, the new mother is admonished to avoid all elements related to cold. Women from the family are present to meet her every need. She is discouraged from getting out of bed except to use the bathroom. Staff, on the other hand, encourages her to get up and take a shower soon after the birth. Have you noticed a reluctance on the part of the Mexican American mothers to shower? A sponge bath may be more appropriate, insuring minimal susceptibility to the effect of "cold air." Providing warm blankets, water at room temperature, warm tea, coffee, or broth, instead of ice water encourages fluid intake and recognizes cultural values and beliefs. In addition warm sitz baths and heat lamps can be used as alternatives to ice packs.

Dietary needs of new mothers focus on "hot" foods to restore balance. You may observe the new mother eating small amounts of hospital food. Does she rely on the family to bring food from home? *Caldo de pollo* (chicken soup), herbal teas, and tortillas provide a balanced meal to meet her needs. The HCP can ask her which foods she prefers to eat and inform the dietary department of these needs. This is a great opportunity to review the hospital's menu. Does it meet the diverse needs of the patient population? It may be time for a change.

Breastfeeding

Ideally, the decision to breastfeed is done prior to delivery. During the prenatal period, educational brochures, videos, and individual/group discussions help to assure that information is provided and questions answered. For many Mexican-American women, breastfeeding begins when the milk comes in, usually on the third day. Colostrum, considered full of nutrients and beneficial to the infant by the professional staff, is considered dirty and stale in the Mexican belief system. This conflict can be a frustrating experience for both mother and staff. The situation may be even more stressful for the new mother when the grandmother, held in high esteem, and to be respected at all times, admonishes her to give the baby a bottle until her milk comes in.

A maternity nurse shared her frustration over a recent experience. She had instructed the mother on the benefits and techniques for breastfeeding and when she left the room, the mother was successfully breast-feeding her infant. She seemed pleased with her ability. Two hours later when the nurse returned, the grandmother was in attendance and the new mother was giving the baby a bottle. Respect for the wisdom and cultural knowledge of the elder had trumped the nurse.

<u>**Reflective exercise**</u>: **Breastfeeding . . .where to start**
1. *What has been your experience with Mexican-American new mothers?*
2. *What works . . . what doesn't?*
3. *How do you include the extended family & especially the grandmother in the process?*
4. *Where do you find common ground with the new mother and family?*

La Cuarentena

La cuarentena is a forty-day birth recuperation period that allows the new mother to care for her infant and regain her strength. It is thought to be a time of increased vulnerability to the mother caused by the imbalance of hot and cold, and by the "unclean" bleeding associated with birth. Restoration of physical balance and purification is accomplished by limited activity, dietary restrictions, and seclusion. Her main focus is to care for her new baby, while everything else is taken care of by the extended family. While this may seem restrictive, it does provide the new mother an opportunity to bond with her infant and show respect to the women in attendance.

Home Health Visits

Home visits, following the birth of the infant, afford an opportunity to view the family within the context of their environment. Listening and observing are key elements during the visit. Some of the frequent concerns heard by home health staff relate to the balance of hot and cold with respect to the infant. Wrapping a baby warmly avoids exposure to cold; however, this may translate into an undue increase of the baby's temperature. How would one reconcile the mother's concern that the infant stay warm with the HCPs knowledge that wrapping the infant in multiple blankets is not healthy? The home health nurse can explain that a great deal of heat is lost through the head, and that wearing a cap will help keep the baby stay warm.

I would like to share with you another related story about the balance of hot and cold. A nurse made a home visit to assess the wellbeing of a two-week-old infant who had recently been hospitalized for gastroenteritis. During the visit, she noted bottles of formula on the windowsill. It was the middle of July and the room was very warm. The mother explained that her husband had put them there before he left for work in the morning so she would not be exposed to the cold when opening the refrigerator door. The milk sat out all day, exposed to the heat from the sun. Acknowledging the mother's cultural beliefs about heat loss was a good first step. The question:

What to do? How does one show respect for another's beliefs in light of the health concerns of the infant? The creative solution was to suggest that the mother dress warmly, with hat, scarf, and gloves before opening the refrigerator. It worked! A win-win for all concerned.

Culture Care Modes & Actions
Mexican – Pregnancy

Caring for the pregnant Mexican-American woman may call us to review our approach and modify our expectations. Using Dr. Leininger's three modes of decision making and action can assist us with integrating the beliefs, values, and health practices ascribed to in the Mexican-American culture. Below are some suggestions. Think about your patient population: what else would you add to the list. It is never straight forward, or the same for every Mexican-American patient, but rather serves as a guide to provide culturally sensitive and competent health care.

Preservation/Maintenance
- Respect for the elderly and those in authority
- Family support
- Rest and avoidance of strenuous activity

Accommodation/Negotiation
- Inclusion of family during the prenatal, intrapartum, and postpartum period
- Visitation of extended family
- Breastfeeding
- Balance of hot and cold

Repatterning/Restructuring
- Diet ~ gestational diabetes

Resources

Al Tajir, G. K., Sulieman, H., Badrinath, P. (2006). Intragroup differences in risk factors for breastfeeding outcomes in a multicultural community. *Journal of Human Lactation.* (22)1, 39-47.

Amerson, R. (2008). Reflections on a conversation with a curandera. *Journal of Transcultural Nursing.* (19)4, 384-387.

Andrews, M. M., Boyle, J. S. (2008). *Transcultural concepts in nursing care.* (5th Ed.).New York: Lippincott Williams & Wilkins.

Barron, F., Hunter, A., Mayo, R., Willoughby, D. (2004). Acculturation and adherence: Issues for healthcare providers working with clients of Mexican origin. *Journal of Transcultural Nursing.* (15)4, 331-337.

Berry, A. B. (1999). Mexican American women's expression of meaning of culturally congruent prenatal care. *Journal of Transcultural Nursing.* (10)3, 202-212.

Berry, A. (2002). Culture care of the Mexican American family. In Leininger, M. M. McFarland, M. R. (Eds.) *Transcultural Nursing: Concepts, Theories, Research & Practice.* (3rd Ed.). New York: McGraw Hill.

Burk, M. E., Wieser, P. C., Keegan, L. (1995). Cultural beliefs and health behaviors of pregnant Mexican-American women: Implications for primary care. *Advances in Nursing Science.* (17)4, 37-52.

Caudle, P. (1993). Providing culturally sensitive health care to Hispanic clients. *Nurse Practitioner.* (18)12. 42-51.

Diversity Resources. (2001). Culture-sensitive health care: Hispanic. Retrieved on November 25, 2001, from: http://www.divrsityresources.com/health2K/health/hispanic.html

Falicov, C.J. (2005). Mexican Families. In McGoldrick, M., Giordano, J. Garcia-Preto, N. (Eds) *Ethnicity & Family Therapy.* (3rd Ed.). New York: Guilford Press

Galanti, G. A. (2004). Caring for Patients from Different Cultures. (3rd Ed.) Philadelphia: University of Pennsylvania Press.

Gill, S. L., Reifsnider, E., Lucke, J. F. (2007). Effects of support on the initiation and duration of breastfeeding. *Western Journal of Nursing Research.* (29)6, 708-723.

Guarnero, P.A. (2005) Mexican Americans. In Lipson, J. G., Dibble, S. L., (Eds.) Culture & Clinical Care. San Francisco CA: UCSF Nursing Press.

Gonzalez, E. W., Owen, D. C., Christina, M., Esperat, R. (2008). Mexican Americans. In Giger, J. N., Davidhizar, R. E. (Eds). *Transcultural Nursing: Assessments and Interventions*. (5th Ed.) St Louis, MO: Mosby/Elsevier.

Helsel, D., Mochel, M. (2002). Afterbirths in the afterlife: Culture meaning of placenta disposal in a Hmong-American community. *Journal of Transcultural Nursing*. (13)4, 282-286.

Juarbe, T. (1995). Access to health care for Hispanic women: A primary health care perspective. *Nursing Outlook*. (43)1, 23-28.

LaGaná, K. (2003). Come bien, camina y so se preocupe – eat right, walk and do not worry: Selective biculturalism during pregnancy in a Mexican America community. *Journal of Transcultural Nursing*. (14)2, 117-124.

Lauderdale, J. (2008). Transcultural Perspectives in Childbearing. In Andrews, M. M., Boyle, J. S. (Eds). Transcultural Concepts in Nursing. (5th Ed.). New York: Lippincott Williams & Wilkins.

Leininger, M. M. (1991). *Culture care diversity and universality: A theory of nursing*. New York: National League for Nursing Press.

Leininger, M. M., McFarland, M. R. (2002). *Transcultural nursing: Concepts, theories, research and practice*. (3rd Ed.). New York: McGraw-Hill.

Lipson, J., Dibble, S., (2005). Culture & Clinical Care. San Francisco, CA: UCSF Nursing Press.

Posmontier, B., Horowitz, J. A. (2004). Postpartum practices and depression prevalences: Technocentric and ethnokinship cultural perspectives. *Journal of Transcultural Nursing*. (15)1, 34-43.

Shusta, R. M., Levine, D. R., Wong, H. Z., Olson, A. T., Harris, P. R. (2008). Multicultural Law Enforcement: Strategies for Peacekeeping in a Diverse Society. (4th Ed.) New Jersey: Pearson, Prentice Hall.

Siatkowski, A. A. (2007). Hispanic acculturation: A concept analysis. *Journal of Transcultural Nursing*. (18)4, 316-323.

Staisak, D. (1991). Culture care theory with Mexican Americans in an urban context. In Leininger, M. M. (Ed.). *Culture care diversity & universality: A theory in nursing*. New York: National League for Nursing Press.

Spector, R. (2009). *Cultural diversity in health and illness*. (7th Ed.), New Jersey: Pearson/Prentice Hall.

U.S Census (2007). Language Use in the United States: 2007. American Community Survey Reports. Retrieved June 19, 2020. www.cenus.gov

Wisneski, L. A., Anderson, L. (2005). *The Scientific Basis of Integrative Medicine*. New York: CRC Press.

Zoucha, R. (1998). The experiences of Mexican Americans receiving professional nursing care: An ethnonursing study. *Journal of Transcultural Nursing*. (9)2, 34-44.

Zoucha, R., Purnell, L. D. (2003). People of Mexican Heritage. In Purnell, L. D., Paulanka, B. J. (Eds). *Transcultural Health Care: A Culturally Competent Approach*. Philadelphia: F. A. Davis.

Zoucha, R., Zamarripa, C. (2008). People of Mexican Heritage. In Purnell, L. D., Paulanka, B. J. (Eds). Transcultural Health Care: A Culturally Competent Approach. (3rd Ed) Philadelphia: F. A. Davis.

You're in America Now! . . . Challenges in The Workplace
(Filipino)

11

Imelda and Lourdes giggle as they walk towards the desk. Although the diminutive nurses look like sisters, they don't link arms any more as they walk, having been cautioned that "it's just not done" in Des Moines. They don't seem to notice Genevieve's glower at them or perhaps they just ignore her. Genevieve has been on duty since 5:30 that morning and the two nurses assume that her frown is due to overwork – a natural thought, especially since the stocky red-faced nurse always seems to look either angry or morose.

Imelda has just replaced Mrs. Swanson's feeding tube and it has reminded her of a story about hummingbirds; she can't wait to tell Lourdes. Even though they had never seen a real hummingbird at home in the Philippines, Imelda has several that visit her feeder by the front door of the apartment. Bright red heads.

"Ito umaga any îbon," she begins.

Genevieve speaks up loudly, in terse English. "Let us all in on the story, why don't you?"

Lourdes shrugs. She can wait for the punch line; break is just ten minutes away.

"Oh, and girls, we have too many patients at the moment to take time out for coffee and sweets. I need you both to finish up with the ledger. Quickly."

"Yes, Miss Genevieve," Imelda and Lourdes burble brightly. They look down in unison.

Neither of the young nurses appears ruffled, though that has been the intent of the reprimand. Nursing in this country is so businesslike, so lacking in true charity, but they are doing their jobs as they see fit, focusing on the comfort of the patient, always smiling when someone in their charge

129

addresses them. Poor old Mr. Kilmer really needs loving attention, not just a brusk change of his bed linen.

"Maybe I'll go see what he needs before I worry about writing down any details," Lourdes muses. "He doesn't have a daughter like me to make sure he's settled well. That ledger, with all its medical hieroglyphics, will have to wait."

Challenges in the workplace

Changes in the work environment are challenging. In this chapter we look at the recruitment of foreign HCPs, specifically *Filipino nurses. The healthcare link between the Philippines and the United States is not new. This link between the two countries began in 1898 when the Philippines were ceded to the United States following the Spanish American War. From 1945 to 1990, thousands of Filipino nurses emigrated to the United States.

*There is no "F" in the indigenous Tagalog language. While the term Pilipino may be used interchangeably with Filipino, for this chapter we will use *Filipino*. Dula Pacqiao (2003 p. 138) indicates the term *Pilipino* is generally used to distinguish indigenous identity and for nationalistic empowerment.

From a historical perspective . . .

The history of the Philippines includes colonization by China, Indonesia, Malaysia, and India. Each contributed to the influence of the cultural heritage of the Filipino people. In 1521 the Spaniards conquered and colonized the Philippine Islands and renamed it *Las Isla de Filipinas* in honor of King Phillip II. Spain occupied the country for three hundred years and introduced their customs and cultural traditions to the people during that time. In 1898 the islands were ceded to the United States in accordance with the Paris Treaty. The name was changed to the Philippines and the influence of American culture on democracy, education, and healthcare began.

In the early 1900s missionaries and medical providers arrived to establish nursing programs and hospitals. Their goal was to serve as collaborators between the United States and the Philippines and to provide educational opportunities for those working in the healthcare field. During that same era, other groups such as the Daughters of the American Revolution and the Catholic Scholarship Fund sponsored individuals to come to the United Sates for training.

A study done in 1920 found that lack of sanitation and insufficient healthcare were contributing factors to the poor health of the people in the Philippines. In 1922 Alice Fitzgerald, an American nurse with international experience, was commissioned by the Rockefeller Foundation to introduce public health nursing to the nursing programs in the Philippines. After meeting with people in the field and visiting healthcare facilities, she proposed five major reform measures.

- Create a central school for nurses
- Establish a league of nursing education
- Organize a national nursing association
- Study and revise state registration laws and examination methods for nurses
- Simplify and standardize nurse training school methods

Brush, B. L. (1995 p. 544)

She was organizing the "American way." Many of the schools were headed by American-born or American trained nurses. As Brush states in her article, "the presence of American leadership in conjunction with a western nursing curriculum confirmed Fitzgerald's confidence that the students would be well trained." (p. 546) During times of high unemployment in the Philippines, coupled with a nursing shortage in the United States, Filipino nurses were recruited to fill the void. Today, as in the early 1900s, nurses in the Philippines are educated according to western standards. So why does there seem to be a conflict in our scenario? One's cultural values, beliefs, and biases influence nursing care practices. Conflict can occur when these are different from those of coworkers in the host country.

Cultural ways we express ourselves

How we see a situation, perceive a need, or resolve a problem is culturally based. In the vignette, Genevieve sees it one way, while Imelda and Lourdes see it another. They attribute Genevieve's frustration to being overworked. Their focus is on the comfort of the patient, not the paperwork. Differing perspectives. Steeped in the Spanish and the Asian cultural values of family, hierarchy, and comfort care, Imelda and Lourdes incorporate this into their work environment. In her research titled Culture Care of Philippine and Anglo-American Nurses in a Hospital Context, Zenaida Splanger (1991) identifies Philippine-American cultural values.

Filipino Cultural Values & Beliefs
- Family unity and closeness
- Respect for elder/authority
- "Leave one-self to God"
- Obligations to sociocultural ties
- Hot-Cold beliefs
- Use of Folk foods and practices
- Religion valued

The value of family and closeness assures support, emotionally and financially, for Filipino nurses who come to live and work in the United States. It is this reassurance that one is not alone, and that resources are readily available within the Filipino community. Family include grandparents, aunts, uncles, and those who are not "blood" related, yet are considered part of the group. Interdependence is woven throughout this network of extended family. *Utang Na Loob* or the "give and take," also referred to as a "debt of honor," refers to the mutual reciprocity along with a sense of gratitude for the favors received from others. Another term used, *bayanihani*, translates into cooperation and a willingness to help others. In the healthcare setting, this value may be a part of the Filipino nurses' belief that assisting one another with patient care is expected (Spangler 1991, Pacquiao 2003). This may conflict with the Anglo-American value of independence, which translates into getting one's work done in a timely manner without assistance.

Avoiding conflict . . . showing respect
Respect for and deference to authority and those who are elderly is a highly held value in the Filipino culture. This is shown by bowing to an elder with hands together, avoiding disagreement, and remaining quiet. Leaders are expected to be followed and are believed to make decisions that are in the best interest of the group. Imelda and Lourdes show respect for Genevieve when they smile and lower their heads in response to her request. Listed below are some terms that relate to respect for elders and authority and avoidance of conflict. Spangler (1991) lists other terms used to connote the value of culture including:

- **Pakikisama:** maintain smooth relationships
- **Amor propio:** save face and self esteem
- **Hiya:** avoid shame

132

These values, as seen through the eyes of the Filipino nurse, promote smooth relationships. One saves face and possible shame through avoidance of conflict especially in a public setting such as the hospital. The American value of openly confronting a situation is in contrast to the Filipino belief of maintaining *pakikisama* ~ the importance of "getting along with others at all costs."

In the Filipino culture, the use a third party or a "go between" helps resolve conflict without losing face. Imelda or Lourdes may enlist the help of a colleague to intercede on their behalf. Recently, an Anglo-American nurse shared with me that "in her opinion," they, the Filipino staff, should just learn to do it "our way." I suggested that possibly an incorporation of the value of maintaining smooth relationships could be an option for staff as well.

Reflective exercise: Responding . . .
1. *Is it difficult for you to remain quiet when a conflict arises?*
2. *Does maintaining smooth relationships supersede responding verbally when there is a difference of opinion?*
3. *Would you prefer to use an intermediary instead of a "face to face" discussion?*
4. *Where do you find common ground with Imelda and Lourdes?*

Communication . . .

In the Filipino culture, the value of showing respect, maintaining smooth relationships, and saving face are reflected in their verbal and nonverbal communication. The Filipino may appear quiet and reserved which may be interpreted as shy to an outsider. The desire to show respect is demonstrated with the avoidance of an overt expression. Requests are made politely, and behavior is influenced by the age, gender, or social position of each person. Usually soft spoken, words take into account setting, circumstances, or ideas. Personal feelings are not openly expressed and can be related to the importance of *pakikisama*. In addition, a "hesitant yes" may really mean "no." What does the body language say? Silence may be used as a sign of respect or to convey a "no" response.

Conversations with family and friends can be loud, expressive, and animated. Within the Filipino community, nonverbal communication is intuitive and overt, but minimal with outsiders. A smile or a nod will convey a message rather than words. Eye contact is used sparingly in conversations with the elderly and those in authority. It helps to protect oneself from "losing face" or respect. Touch is valued within the Filipino community. It is common for women to walk arm in arm. At many of my seminars, it is the Filipino women who share their story about receiving strange looks from people as they walked "arm in arm." Two Filipino nurses laughed as they shared their story. Even though they have lived in the United States for twenty years, they have to remind themselves not to walk arm in arm when out in public or at the hospital.

Language in the workplace

Have you ever tried to learn a second language? As a child that would have been easier . . . but as an adult it takes great courage, determination, and time. Speaking from experience, the book learning part in a controlled classroom setting is easy compared with "real" conversation in the clinical area. I remember sitting with a group in Cuernavaca, Mexico, during one of my Spanish immersion programs when the intensity and the speed of the conversation suddenly increased. I found myself "lost in translation." I relied on the "nod and smile" routine, which translates into "I don't have a clue what you are saying, but I will act like I understand because I don't want you to think I am stupid."

Learning a second language not only takes an incredible amount of time and effort, but it uses different facial muscles, which adds to the exhaustion. Stress affects the ability to remember, thus one may revert back to his or her primary language: English, Spanish, Tagalog, Russian, Chinese, or another. Clinical areas can be filled with tension, and HCPs from foreign countries may rely on their primary language to convey a message.

Language other than English in the hospital or clinical arena has generated a healthy debate. For English-only speakers, this may create distrust or uncertainty. The concern seems to center on being "left out" or thinking your coworker is making negative comments about you. Genevieve, concerned that Imelda and Lourdes' conversation was about her, interjected a terse comment to them "let us all in on the story, why don't you?" The story is about a hummingbird, but Genevieve doesn't speak Tagalog so she would not know this.

In the workplace setting it is important to have guidelines, expectations, and policies in place that clearly define when it is acceptable to use a language other than English. English-only patients may be concerned about what is being said. In order to provide respect and a sense of security for the patient, the HCPs should refrain from using their primary language in front of an English-speaking patient. When the HCP, fluent in another language, converses with patients who speak for example, Tagalog, Spanish or Russian, this promotes understanding, alleviates concerns and establishes trust and rapport with both the patient and the family.

Reflective excersize: In another language . . .
1. *Have you ever been in a situation in which you did not understand the language being spoken?*
2. *How did you feel?*
3. *Did you pretend to understand?*
4. *In your workplace, what languages are spoken by your colleagues?*
5. *By your patients?*
6. *Are there policies that address language in the workplace?*

Time is of the essence . . . don't think so!

The past-time orientation of the Filipino people is directly attributable to the influence of the Asian and the Spanish cultures. Respect is shown to ancestors and those who have recently died. Funerals are lavish events followed by nine days of prayers and family gatherings. A year anniversary completes the cycle with a visit to the grave site bringing flowers and favorite stories and song.

Time is viewed as relative to the present situation as well. The present moment cannot be "recaptured" at a later time. This may translate into being late for an appointment because something unforeseen happened which needed immediate attention. Usually for work or business, one arrives on time. For the Filipino HCPs, taking the time to listen to the patient and providing comfort may delay "getting work done on time" and may appear to coworkers as an inability to set priorities and organize their time.

The lack of concern for the future embraces the concept of *bahala na* or God willing, a fatalistic approach to life. When outside or supernatural forces are in control, one learns to accept unquestionably what life or death brings. However, there is a strong family commitment to the future through education. Children are expected to do well in school, which translates to a secure economic status. Parents care for the children (present orientation), and the children are expected to care for them in their old age (future orientation).

Families

There is a strong sense of family, which is hierarchal, patriarchal, and extended. The father is acknowledged as the head of the household, yet the mother may hold an equal position. The greater the educational and economic level of the family, the more likely they are to have an egalitarian approach to decision making and parenting. Traditional roles for women, such as caregiver and homemaker are changing as more enter the workforce. Grandparents, held in high esteem, assume the responsibility of care giving and occasionally the discipline of the children.

Children are valued. They are raised in a highly protective environment that includes limitations on activities and socialization. They are taught an an early age to show respect and deference for their elders and not to question decisions. Obedience, avoiding direct confrontations, and refraining from showing emotions are clear expectations set by parents.

Healthcare practices

The influence of the Four Humors and the belief in the hot/cold theory was brought to the Philippines from China and Spain. It is very much a part of their health beliefs and practices today as well as western medicine. Mal aire, or bad wind, is thought to be another cause of illness. Exposure to a sudden cold draft may be the cause of a cold, fever, or upper respiratory infection The cultural value of *Bahala na ~ God Willing*, leaving in God's hands, promotes an external locus of control, thus the belief that illness and health are not determined or affected by the patient's actions or decisions. Health is the result of balance in one's life, physically, mentally, and spiritually. This holistic approach underscores the essence of cause and cure. Good nutrition, exercise, rest and maintaining smooth relationships with others are ways that promote health.

Illness aligns with supernatural or magioreligious beliefs as well. Having negative thoughts about the dead may cause evil spirits to enter the body. For some, there is a belief that certain people have extraordinary powers to cast spells causing illness. Mental illness is thought to be due to an external cause such as witchcraft, soul loss, or intrusion of an evil spirit. Protection from harmful spirits is assured by wearing amulets, reciting prayers, and seeking the advice from a folk healer. Healing rituals include prayer sessions, exorcism, herbs, and massage.

Treatment may come from a variety of sources in addition to those already mentioned. The sick person will stoically attempt to care for him or herself. If there is no improvement, he or she will seek the advice of family or folk healers such as curers or hilots. Curers diagnose an illness by taking the pulse and determining whether it is "hot" or "cold." Treatment brings balance. The Hilot provides healing through prayer, herbal medicine, and massage and/or manipulation of bones and body tissue. Some of the treatments include hitting with malongi leaves to ward off evil spirits, anointing with oils, and holding family prayer sessions. Religious practices are very much a part of the healing process as well. Patients may present to an appointment with visible signs of their belief such as wearing a scapula or cross or holding rosary beads in their hands. Asking for forgiveness from someone is thought to have restorative properties well.

The caring role in the family is designated mainly to women. The role of the sick person is clear. They are to be pampered and taken care of until recovery. They are not expected to "do for themselves." This may be in direct conflict with the western theory that promotes self-care. Caution should be taken not to be intrusive or demanding of the patient, but to find common ground in developing a plan of care. Physicians are held in high esteem, thus the patient may be hesitant to question the plan of care (*pakikisama*). In addition, if the patient is not following the plan, then the HCP needs to find out if this is due to *bahala na* or a lack of understanding on the part of the patient and family.

Reflective exercise: Beliefs about . . .
1. *Do you believe that illness can be caused by supernatural means?*
2. *Do your religious beliefs help you get well?*
3. *In what way are your health beliefs similar to the Filipino patient?*
4. *In what ways are they different?*
5. *Where do you find common ground?*

*   *   *   *

Do you have more in common with Filipino nurses than you first thought? Your goal to provide quality patient care is synonymous with the goals of the Filipino nurses. Your differences may center on the interpretation of beliefs and values of the Filipino and American culture. Realizing that there is more common ground than first thought, compromise and collaboration invite new perspectives in patient care. Through this process we create a welcoming environment that is open to discussion and resolution of issues that arise in our healthcare settings.

Culture Care Modes & Actions
Filipino – Multicultural Workforce

Preservation/Maintenance
- Family loyalty and extended family
- Respect for elderly and those in authority
- Comfort care
- Nursing as vocation

Accommodation/Negotiation
- Use eye contact sparingly with those in authority
- Save face ~ Avoid shame
- Present-time orientation
- Primary language with Tagalog-speaking patients and at breaks

Restructure/Repattern
- Primary language around colleagues and English-speaking-only patients

Resources

Andrews, M. M., Boyle, J. S. (2008). *Transcultural concepts in nursing care*. (5th Ed.).New York: Lippincott Williams & Wilkins.

Andrews, M. M. (1998). Transcultural perspectives in nursing administration. *Journal of Nursing Administration*. (28)11, 30-38.

Brush, B. L. (1995). The Rockefeller agenda for American/Philippines nursing relations. *Western Journal of Nursing Research*. (17)5, 540-555.

Cantos, A., Rodriguez, D. M., de Guzman, C. P. (2005) Filipinos. In Lipson, J. G., Dibble, S. L., (Eds.) Culture and Clinical Care. San Francisco CA: UCSF Nursing Press.

Edraline, M. D. (2007). The Philippines: Filipino history, culture and heritage. Retrieved on August 2, 2007, from http://inic.utexas.edu/asnic/countries/philippines/philippines.html

Falicov, C. J. (2005). Mexican Families. In McGoldrick, M., Giordano, J. Garcia-Preto, N. (Eds) *Ethnicity & Family Therapy*. (3rd Ed.). New York: Guilford Press

Galanti, G. A. (2004). *Caring for Patients from Different Cultures*. (3rd Ed.) Philadelphia: University of Pennsylvania Press.

Gamble, D. A. (2002). Filipino nurse recruitment as a staffing stategy. *Journal of Nursing Administration*. (32)4, 175-177.

Hayne, A. N., Gerhardt, C., Davis, J. (2009). Filipino nurses in the United States: Recruitment, retention, occupational stress and job satisfaction. *Journal of Transcultural Nursing*. 1-10.

Kenton, S. B., Valentine, D. (1997). *Crosstalk: Communicating in a Multicultural Workplace*. New Jersey: Prentice Hall.

Leininger, M. M. (2002). Philippine Americans and culture care. In Leininger, M. M., McFarland, M. R. (Eds). *Transcultural Nursing: Concepts, Theories, Research & Practice*. (3rd Ed.). New York: McGraw Hill.

Leininger, M. M., McFarland, M. R. (2002). *Transcultural nursing: Concepts, theories, research and practice*. (3rd Ed.). New York: McGraw-Hill.

Ludwig-Beymer, P. (2008). Creating Culturally Competent Organizations. In Andrews, m.M., Boyle, J. S. (Eds). *Transcultural Cocepts in Nursing Care*. (5th Ed.). New York: Lippincott. Williams & Wilkins

Pacquiao, D. F (2008). People of Filipino Heritage. In Purnell, L.D., Paulanka B. J. (3rd Ed). *Transcultural Health Care: A Culturally Competent Approach*. Philadelphia: F. A. Davis.

Root, M.P.P. (2005). Filipino families. In McGoldrick, M. M., Giordano, J., Garcia-Preto, N. (Eds.) *Ethnicity & Family Therapy*. (3rd Ed.). New York: The Guilford Press.

Spangler, Z D. (1991). Culture care of Philippine and Anglo-American nurses in a hospital setting. In Leininger, M.M. (Ed.). *Culture care diversity & universality: A theory in nursing*. New York: National League for Nursing Press.

Spector, R. (2009). *Cultural diversity in health and illness*. (7th Ed.), New Jersey: Pearson/Prentice Hall.

Vance, A.R. (2008). Filipino Americans. In Giger, J. N., Davidhizar, R. E. (Eds). *Transcultural Nursing: Assessments and Interventions*. (5th Ed.) St Louis, MO: Mosby/Elsevier.

I'm Not Leaving the Room . . .

(Jewish Orthodox)

12

But first . . . a bit of history

From the destruction of the Jewish temple in 70 CE (Common Era), to the Spanish Inquisition of 1478, to the pogroms (anti-Jewish riots and murders) in Russia and Eastern Europe in the mid 19th century, to the Holocaust during World War II, Jewish people have been subject to persecution. The riots and massacre by the Romans in 70 CE led to the great diaspora of the Jewish people to diverse parts of the globe. Being "Jewish" is not considered to be a specific race, therefore, but rather a people and a religion.

Jewish immigrants to the United States came from all parts of the world. Sephardic Jews, from Brazil, were the first to settle in New Amsterdam in the mid 1600s. The early part of the nineteenth century saw a large emigration from Germany following persecution in Bavaria. In the later part of the century Eastern European Jews came from Russia, Poland, and Romania. Most recently the largest emigration has come from the former Soviet Republic.

Jewish beliefs are based on the tenets found in the Torah (five books written by Moses) and the Talmud (the Rabbinic code). In the Middle Ages, these served to govern religious behavior, rituals during birth and death, preparation of food, and the proper clothing. Because of the strict adherence to the commandments and tenets of the Torah, Jewish culture and world view segregated them from the general population. There are now four branches: Orthodox, Reform, Conservative, and Reconstructivist. The Orthodox Jew maintains strict adherence to the law and the commandments. The Reform movement started in Germany in the nineteenth century when there was less isolation from the general public and includes more integration with the general population. The Reform Jew generally holds a flexible viewpoint of Jewish law. The Conservative branch, thought to be somewhere between Orthodox and Reform, started around the same time in Germany. Believing the Reform Jew was too modern, the Conservatives, while preserving the core values of Judaism, interpreted the tenets strictly based on the society and the times. The Reconstructivist branch, an outgrowth of the Conservative movement, holds a humanistic approach and follows the law because of its cultural value. (Giger and Davidhizar 2008)

For many Jewish people, illness or imminent death is a time to explore one's relationship with God. As HCPs, we are not always aware of Jewish healthcare practices, especially the differences between Orthodox, Reform, Conservative, and Reconstructivist. The focus of this chapter addresses those areas of commonality within each sect as well as end-of-life beliefs and practices in the Jewish faith and tradition.

And now to the story . . . I am not leaving the room!

"Stanley looks so peaceful there, even with all the tubes," Lynn Rubenstein thought. "I hope we won't have another episode like last night. Those nurses are so insensitive. I couldn't believe they actually wanted me to leave my husband of fifty-five years all alone while they jolted his heart. Stanley has such a big heart too. They just don't know what a love he's been. Well, except for when he's so positive about something and needs to raise his voice to convince me. I'm sure glad he signed that form about no organ donations though. He's way too old to have his kidneys save someone else's life, of course, but the idea that some one not of the blood might get some part of him is just too dreadful."

Stanley Rubenstein did look peaceful too. His breathing was only a little labored and, given the sleep apnea he'd had for most of their married life, that was a good sign. His heart was giving up though; the Supreme Physician was calling him home, no matter how good the care was in ICU here at Mass General.

Lynn Rubenstein had met her husband at Temple Beth-el sixty years before. When she discovered that Stanley was two years through law school even though he was just nineteen, she knew he was the one for her. She'd heard of the family too, of course. Her own family had just moved to Boston after living in New York for generations, but the Rubensteins were

Old Boston; good blood lines. After all these years, she still felt a bit off balance here, and the hospital was making it worse.

"I wish the family hadn't decided on Mass General. A good Jewish hospital would have staff that understood. In this one, even the one rabbi is supposed to be there for all of us whether we're Reform, Conservative, or Orthodox. That fellow who came in yesterday had the tiniest yamulke I'd ever seen; didn't look very pious to me."

Anna and Suzette came bustling into the tiny room. Mrs. Rubenstein had been able to get a single for Stanley, but it was still a "crawl space," as she put it when talking to her friend Naomi Sills. The nurses fiddled with the urine sac and the tubes, glancing at the various monitors hooked up to the pale form in the bed.

"We're going to have to be alone for a minute or two, Mrs. Rubenstein. The doctor will be here shortly and your husband needs to have our full attention while we prep him. The waiting room is just down the hall."

The two nurses braced themselves for a fight. For some reason, Mrs. Rubenstein just wouldn't leave her husband, no matter how many years they'd been together. You'd think a few minutes wouldn't be too much to ask. Yesterday, they'd had to get extra help from an orderly to escort her out.

"Jesus, Mary, and Joseph," Suzette whispered.

*   *   *   *

Jewish law dictates that a person is not left alone when the possibility of death looms. This law is strictly adhered to by the Orthodox Jew. It may not be followed by the Reform, Conservative or Reconstructionist, though each may display similar behavior relative to their cultural knowledge of Law. Asking family to leave the room adds a great deal of stress to an already difficult situation. It is the belief that when the person dies, the spirit departs from the body and if no one is present, the soul will feel alone and desolate. (Sperling 1968 p. 604)

Cultural Beliefs and Values

The importance of maintaining respect for the religious beliefs and practices of Judaism are central to the cultural values and beliefs of Jewish-American culture. Research done in various urban communities between 1975 and 1991 by Dr. Leininger and other transcultural nurses indicate there are variations within the four branches as well as intergenerational

143

ones. Values held strongly by first and second generation Jewish-Americans may not hold the same weight for succeeding generations.

Jewish Orthodox Cultural Values & Beliefs

- Centrality of family with patriarchal rule and mother care (although this is changing with increased acculturation to a more egalitarian situation)
- Support of education and intellectual achievements
- Maintenance of the continuity of Jewish heritage
- Generosity and charity to the arts, music, and community service
- Achievement of success (financial and educational)
- Persistence and persuasion
- Closeness and shared suffering
- Enjoyment of the arts, music, and religious rituals

Leininger (1991, p. 366)

Each of these cultural values and beliefs offers insight into the importance of heritage, tradition, support, and family. The belief by Jews that they are God's chosen people includes a history of persecution, thus suffering may be seen as part of life itself, something to be endured. A well-known Yiddish saying, *Shver zu zein a yid* ("It's tough to be a Jew") accompanied by a sigh suggests that there may be pride in suffering (Rosen, Weltman 1996 p. 616). As a HCP you may notice that complaints may be followed by a sigh. It is important to understand the message and not to stereotype.

> **Reflective exercise: Cultural beliefs and values**
> 1. *Have you observed these beliefs and practices with your Jewish patients?*
> 2. *How are your beliefs different from theirs?*
> 3. *Where do you find common ground?*
> 4. *Knowing this information, how could you use this to meet the needs of your Jewish patients?*

Family

In Jewish societies, the family is central. As with many family structures, the role of the father as the breadwinner and the mother as the homemaker is changing as well. For some Jewish families this may also be dependent on the specific religious affiliation. The more Orthodox, the more structured, the greater adherence to tenets such as the father's obligation to educate his children in Judaism, to teach his sons a trade, and to provide his daughters with the means to make them marriageable. The mother's role is to keep a Jewish home and raise the children. (Selekman 2004 p. 236). The feminist movement in the 1970s laid the groundwork for Jewish women to seek careers, study the Torah, and (since 1972) become rabbis. The value of family and children, coupled with the value of intellect, education, and financial success, may make it stressful to balance all aspects.

Children are highly valued and are to be protected, although some literature suggests that independence is encouraged. While overprotectiveness may be related to the days of fear in Eastern Europe, independence may be seen as an acculturation to American values. Respect for elders as acknowledged by the commandments, the injunction to "honor thy father and thy mother," instills in the child the importance of social relationships not only with parents but also with teachers, extended family, and rabbis. Seen as the future of the Jewish community, children are encouraged to learn about their history, traditions, and religion. Education is highly valued and respected as well as being something to strive for at an early age; achievement and success validate the love and hard work of the parents. It is important for the HCP to inquire as to the religious beliefs of the family so as to address the needs in a manner that is respectful of the individual patient.

Reflective exercise: Family
1. *In what ways was your family different?*
2. *In what ways similar?*
3. *What was your family's view of education?*
4. *How would you approach the family to assure understanding?*

Communication

Jewish communication is expressive, using both inflections in the voice and gestures to convey a message. Jews can be quite verbal about their feelings. Emphasis on certain words used in Yiddish and now in English may change the meaning of the message. An example given by Enid Schwartz, author of Jewish Americans in Giger and Davidhizar's book, *Transcultural Nursing*, illustrates how this occurs using the phrase "Him you trust." "*Him* you trust?" versus "Him you *trust*?"

145

The first questions the person's judgment, while the second implies that anyone who would trust the character of such a scoundrel must be an idiot. (2004 p. 595) Humor, another frequently used format in conversation, is thought to be a way to cope with the difficulties in life or the hostility and persecution faced by previous generations.

Some dialog used in Jewish families may seem critical and cynical, but this method of communication is sometimes used to get a response or a reaction from a family member. In this situation, the HCP may feel uncomfortable with what seems to be apparent hostility, but from the family member's perspective, it may be the way care is shown, encouraging him or her to voice the real concern. Active listening on the part of the HCP leads to a better understanding of what the patient is expressing.

> **Reflective exercise: Communication**
> 1. *How does your style of communication compare/contrast?*
> 2. *Do loud and expressive people make you feel uncomfortable?*
> 3. *Does humor help you cope with difficult situations?*

Touch and Modesty and Space

Jewish beliefs about the value of touch vary according to the branch of Judaism to which they are affiliated. Other than hands-on care, touch may seem intrusive and cause stress for the patient. Hasidic Jewish men, members of an ultra-Orthodox branch, are only permitted to touch their wives. Handshakes are not welcome from women. If uncertain about the branch of affiliation, you should wait for the patient to extend a tactile sign for a handshake before extending your hand. Modesty is highly valued by both Orthodox Jewish men and women.

Personal and social space are valued by the Jewish people during illness. Having family members close at hand addresses the cultural value of support and assurance in uncertain times. During hospitalization of a loved one, family members provide comfort and may be the voice of the patient when he or she is unable to speak for him or herself.

Time . . . then and now

Past, present, and future orientation are all part of the Jewish tradition. The past is the story "never to forget" the experiences of the Holocaust and the Pogroms. During a wedding ceremony, the past is remembered when the groom breaks a glass to acknowledge the destruction of the Jewish temple during the Roman invasion. The past is also to remember a loved one on the anniversary of his or her death. A candle is lit and the group recites Kaddish, a prayer that praises God and affirms one's faith.

Present day orientation focuses on doing good deeds now. Consistent with the Jewish cultural values, volunteering in programs for the less fortunate, participating in social movements, and promoting the arts and education are held in high esteem. Current problems that go unresolved may caused anxiety about the future.

The Jewish future is synonymous with children and education. Both tradition (Torah) and academics (secular education) are valued. College preparation begins in early childhood in hopes of securing a good life. Worrying about the future, especially during illness, reflects the potential impact of the current illness on the family.

Healthcare and Religious Practices

Religion and healthcare practices may go hand in hand. Maintaining health and wellbeing (body and soul) is a prescribed religious requirement. Tenets of the Torah focus on hygiene, exercise, proper diet, and prevention of disease. The Orthodox Jew's wellbeing and health are more dependent on following the tenets than are other members of the Reform, Conservative, or Reconstructivist branches.

Jewish Americans are knowledgeable about preventative healthcare and are usually up-to-date on the most current information. The physician, seen as a divine mediator between the individual and God, is held in high esteem. It is the responsibility of the patient to seek care when ill and to be an active participant with the physician to develop a plan of care. Family members support and aid in this process to assure the plan is followed. Those who have a connection with healthcare providers in the medical field may encourage the individual to get other opinions before making a final decision. Acknowledging the inclusive nature of the family unit and the Jewish community, the HCP can collaborate with the patient to assure understanding.

When the individual becomes ill, the whole family mobilizes and suffers with and for that person. A patient's expressive verbalization of the symptoms of discomfort and pain is expected and accepted as a way to communicate needs. This expression of distress, in and of itself, may provide relief to the individual. If the patient is unable to tell the HCP about the pain, a family member may be the voice for him or her in getting the attention of the HCP.

Religious practices, such as prayers, observation of the Sabbath, and of the kosher must be considered during hospitalization. The Orthodox Jew prays three times a day as well as before and after meals. Providing water for washing at these times is essential. Some degree of moderation may be used by the remaining three branches. The Jewish Sabbath, which begins before sundown on Friday and ends after sunset on Saturday, is strictly adhered to by the Orthodox Jew. Answering the phone, using the call light, cutting toilet paper, and turning on a light are not allowed. An alternative plan by the HCP, insuring frequent assessments, must be in place.

Kosher means "fit to eat" and is defined rigidly as to the types of food that may be eaten as well as the preparation of such food. Pork and pork products, shellfish (fish with fins and tails are permitted), and birds of prey are avoided. Milk and meat products are not to be mixed. Diet can range from very strict adherence to occasional compliance. In the hospital setting, a kosher meal is served on a paper plate and contains sealed plastic utensils. If the discharge plan from the hospital includes home health, meetings with the patient, family, and home health staff prior to discharge help to assure understanding of dietary needs and restrictions.

Seriously ill or dying

If the patient is seriously ill or dying, the nursing staffs' responsibility to care for the patient may not align with the family's need to be present. Being with the seriously ill or dying person is a family affair, and members take turns holding vigil. As mentioned earlier, the commandment that a dying person is never left alone is a strongly held belief. Had Suzette and Anna been aware of the cultural beliefs, values, and health practices of the Rubensteins, there seemingly insensitivity could have been avoided. In what ways could we facilitate this process, thus decreasing the anxiety and distress of the family and the relatives?

Asking about the patient's religious beliefs and practices, end of life directives, and expectations of the family during the admissions assessment might make a difference. A collaborative approach to involving the family, rabbi, physician, social worker, and nursing personnel would facilitate understanding and respect for the cultural belief and practices. Family members expect to be vocal participants in this process.

If death is near, Jewish law dictates that the patient be told; but as several sources suggest, there are passages in the Torah that offer a different perspective. On the one hand, informing the person allows time to get his or her affairs in order, while on the other, telling the individual may remove all hope and may hasten death. Family conferences are an excellent venue for discussion about end of life issues.

The sanctity of life, along with the imperative need to preserve life, is a tenet of the cultural belief system of the Jewish patient. Nothing must be done to hasten death. New treatments that artificially extend life are not implemented. If, for example, the use of a mechanical system such as a ventilator delays death rather than prolonging life, it should not be used.

Reflective exercise: Health and Religious rituals
1. *Does your assessment tool identify religious and cultural needs?*
2. *Do you hold family conferences?*
3. *What are your beliefs about artificial means to sustain life?*
4. *How does this contrast with the beliefs of the Jewish patient?*
5. *Where do you find common ground?*

End of life

Keeping constant vigil at the bedside of a dying patient shows respect for the person as he or she passes from this life. Believing in a direct link with God, the patient may be encouraged by family members to ask for forgiveness and to say the Shema confirming his or her belief. Prior to death, it is prudent for the HCP to inquire of the family which rituals and practices will be followed. When death does occur, the eldest son or a designate gently closes the eyes and mouth of the deceased, then covers the face with a sheet. The preparation of the body following death also may require specific rituals, and it is imperative that the HCP be aware of the requirements. For the ultra-Orthodox Jew, the deceased is to be placed on a mat on the floor, the feet pointing toward the door, and a lit candle placed near the head. In the traditional branch, the Holy Society known as *Hevrah-Kadisha* (Chevra-Kadisha) may prepare the body for burial.

Funerals usually occur within twenty-four to forty-eight hours after death. It begins with the eldest son or designated individual reciting the *Kaddish*, praising God and reaffirming one's own faith. This prayer is also said three times a day during *Shiva*, a seven-day mourning that follows the burial. During this time mourners are "sitting shiva" (providing comfort and emotional support for family and friends). This activity is usually held at the home of the deceased. People are encouraged to bring charitable gifts. Mirrors are covered in the house during this time. There seem to be a variety of reasons – either it's a traditional folk practice that prevents the spirit from coming back and snatching the mourners to the other side – or it's to decrease the vanity of looking at oneself in the mirror. The bereavement period, eleven months from death, culminates in the dedication ceremony or unveiling ceremony held at the cemetery.

> <u>**Reflective exercise**</u>: **End of Life**
> 1. *What are the end of life rituals in your family . . . your culture . . . your religion?*
> 2. *In what ways are they the same . . . different?*
> 3. *What other cultural groups have a specific number of days for a mourning period?*

Autopsy ~ Organ Donation ~ Transplant

In Judaism, the body must be buried whole. Are there exceptions? Yes and No. It is, in many ways, dependent on the circumstance of the situation. While an autopsy is to be avoided as it is seen as the desecration of the body, there are times when it is allowed.

Dorff (1998) lists three extenuating circumstances:
1. It is required by the law
2. The deceased person has willed it
3. It saves the life of another

The same is true with organ donation and transplant. The desire is to bury the body intact, but if it would save the life of another, then it is permissible. Again, it is in having the opportunity to establish a respectful and collaborative relationship with the family through the process of conferences that many of these decisions can be held prior to the end.

*   *   *   *

We as HCPs have the opportunity to provide care that meets the expectations of patients. In the case of Lynn and Stanley Rubenstein, the importance and value of staying with a family member when the situation is critical exceeds adherence to the request of the nurses. We need to talk with family members throughout the hospital experience and to show flexibility and respect for the differences that may surface. Having a plan of care that incorporates cultural and religious beliefs, values, and practices helps to assure a positive outcome for patient, family, and staff.

Culture Care Modes & Actions
Jewish Orthodox – End of Life

Preservation/Maintenance
- Prayer three times a day
- Kosher meals
- Sabbath rituals
- Modesty

Accommodation/Negotiation
- Allow spouse to remain with the patient
- Family visitation
- Family participation in developing plan of care
- End of life decisions

Resources

Andrews, M. M., Boyle, J. S. (2008). *Transcultural concepts in nursing care*. (5th Ed.).New York: Lippincott Williams & Wilkins.

Austerlic, S. (2009). Culturally humility and compassionate presence at the end of life Retrieved June 20, 2009, from http://www.scu.edu/practicing/focusareas/medical/culturally-competentcare.html

Bonura, D., Fender, M., Roesler, M., Pacquiao, D. (2001). Culturally congruent end-of-life care for Jewish patients and their families. *Journal of Transcultural Nursing*. (12)3, 211-220.

Dennis, J. (1999). Love is as strong as death: Meeting the pastoral needs of the Jewish hospice patient. *American Journal of Hospice & Palliative Care*. (16)4, 598-604.

Jacobs, L. A., Giarelli, E. (2001). Jewish culture, health belief systems, and genetic risk for cancer. *Nursing Forum*. (36)2, 5-13.

Leininger, M. M., McFarland, M. R. (2002). *Transcultural nursing: Concepts, theories, research and practice*. (3rd Ed.). New York: McGraw-Hill.

Purnell, L., Selekman, J. (2008). People of Jewish Heritage. In Purnell, L.D., Paulanka, B.J., (Eds.) *Transcultural Health Care: A Culturally Competent Approach*. (3rd Ed.). Philadelphia, PA: F.A. Davis Company

Rosen, E. J., Weltman, S. F. (2005). Jewish families: An Overview. In McGoldrick, M. M., Giordano, J., Garcia-Preto, N (Eds.) *Ethnicity and Family Therapy* (3rd Ed.) New York: Guilford Press.

Selekman, J. (2004). People of Jewish heritage. In Purnell, L. D., Paulanka, B. J. (Eds.) *Transcutural Health Care: A Culturally Competent Approach*.

Soudakoff, S. A. Jewish funeral and mourning customs. Retrieved on January 4, 2006, from http://www.jdcc.org/sepoct97/doc1.htm

Sperling, A. (1968). Reasons for Jewish Customs and Traditions. New York: Bloch.

Schwartz, E. (2008). Jewish Americans. In Giger, J. N., Davidhizar, R. E. (Eds.) *Transcultural Nursing: Assessment and Intervention*. (5th Ed.). St Louis, MO: Mosby/Elsevier.

The Struggle Never Ends . . . Don't They Understand?
(Bosnian Refugee)

13

Servana was thinking about the forest. The Lyrrina family, her mother's side, had a country home there, in the shade of the pines. Too close, it turned out that summer, too easy to march the men off into the trees. Servana sighed, remembering her dear husband Paul and her ten-year-old son. She couldn't even bring herself to whisper his name. She wiped the tear running down next to her long straight nose.

Her thinking was muddled these days. She was tired from the sleepless nights on her cousin's futon. She was grateful to her cousin, of course, but felt like a burden. She washed the dishes when she could and she tried to keep the futon pushed back into a sofa when she went out. But she could hear them whispering about money from behind the door. Her glossy black hair, which had always been her best feature, was now threaded with gray.

Servana was tired of looking for a job. She needed to find a job that could pay better than the one at Donut Delight; at home she had been a legal secretary, but the laws here were so different. Everything was different in Indiana. Not a forest in sight, just cars.

Servana's accent was thick, another impediment to her ready acceptance in Evansville. Probably speaking with her cousin instead of having a good job where she said more than "how many?" and "glazed or sugar?" exacerbated the problem too. How was she going to help out financially if she was deep-frying donuts all day? How could she find a job that focused on her education and ability, but maybe didn't demand that she be totally fluent in English? The accent here in Indiana was really different from that of her teacher at home in Bosnia. And here, down south in Indiana near Kentucky, it was even harder to understand.

Dominique Fuentes was another issue. Her English was difficult for Servana sometimes, but that wasn't really what bothered her. For some

153

reason her social worker, though clean and polite, kept speaking of her as an immigrant instead of a refugee.

"Did you have your family dragged away from Honduras?" Servana wanted to ask. "Did you choose to come here or were you so frightened that you knew that you just couldn't stay where your family had been murdered?"

There was a part of Servana that resented Dominique for having a real job. She'd heard that the Fuentes family had been here in Indiana for several years and she didn't begrudge others who were trying to make their lives better, but she wanted a choice. She didn't choose to lose her husband and son. She didn't choose to lose her well-paying job or to move from her roomy, well-lit home to the apartment of a distant cousin. Although she'd been part of a minority in Bosnia, as a Christian Croat, here, from her native country, she was even more marginalized.

"At least," Servana thought, "Dominique could call me a refugee; I am just taking refuge here. I can choose that. I choose not to be called "an immigrant."

What is the difference . . . why does it matter?

Immigrants come voluntarily to this country. Refugees enter due to war, genocide, or religious or political persecution. If assured safety and security in their home country, the choice to remain is simple: stay. Both immigrants and refugees are hoping to settle in this country and to establish a good life for themselves and their families. Assimilation is an uphill battle for many. Language is the first and greatest barrier. Inability to speak English limits newcomers in securing employment and hinders their taking advantage of resources.

Immigrants have been coming to the United States for hundreds of years. In 1798 the Founding Fathers passed a law establishing new terminology: nativist and immigrant. They considered themselves nativists and those who came after them immigrants. People continue to come to the United States in search of a "better life," with economic stability. Over one million immigrants enter each year, the majority from Mexico and Asia. Immigrants are required to have a sponsor who assures financial support and/or a job. A criterion for permanent residence (green card) is that the individual does not use any publicly funded programs.

Unlike immigrants, refugees enter under duress. They do not leave their countries of origin voluntarily. Each refugee's experience is unique and personal. Servana, widowed during the ethnic cleansing, suffers the effects of the civil war in Bosnia-Herzegovina. Remembering the brutality,

154

the death of family members and loved ones, rape, and starvation continue to haunt her. Those memories and the years in a refugee camp can never be erased. Post traumatic stress disorder, a result of such an experience, can have paralyzing effects, mentally and physically, when one is trying to adjust to a new country such as the United States.

Today . . . Yesterday

Bosnian and Herzegovina were parts of Yugoslavia, which also included Slovenia, Croatia, Serbia, Montenegro and Macedonia. Following the collapse of communism, Bosnia-Herzegovina was home to Muslims, Eastern Orthodox Serbs and Roman Catholic Croats. In the 1980s Serbian party leader Slobodan Milosevic became the ruler and encouraged the beginnings of Serb nationalism. In 1991, he attempted to gain control of the federal government. Slovenia and Croatia sought independence. The Bosnian people called for a referendum for their independence as well in 1992. What followed was three years of civil war with the Bosnian Serbs focusing on ethnic cleansing – genocide, in other words. The goal was to establish a "pure" Serb republic. Muslims, Croats, and Serbs who were opposed to the "Greater Serbia" were cut off from food, utilities, and communication; to venture outside meant certain death. Terrorizing at the hands of Serbs was a daily experience. People watched family members and loved ones die. Villages were destroyed. They were placed in detention camps only to be tortured, raped, and executed. According to the Center for Balkan Development, more than two hundred and fifty thousand persons died, and millions were deported or forced to flee their homes. Nearly three million people became refugees. Finally, the Dayton Peace Accord was signed in December of 1995.

The effects of war . . .

Top trauma events reported by one group of Bosnian refugees

80% ..... experienced unexpected death of a loved one
74.2% ..... experienced events related to living in a war zone
52% ..... had a loved one survive a life-threatening event
45.5% ..... were threatened to be killed by a stranger
44.4% ..... experienced a natural disaster
41.8% ..... saw a stranger attack someone else
31.5% ..... had been robbed or present during a robbery

Craig et al. (2007)

Depression and anxiety, along with the diagnosis of post traumatic stress disorder (PTSD), are everyday challenges for some refugees. PTSD is associated with those who experience significant trauma that includes high levels of violence, along with a sense of constant fear and helplessness to change the situation. Symptoms can include re-experiencing a violent or traumatic event and numbing sensations as well as hyperarousal symptoms. Each of these may lead to sleep disorders, inability to concentrate, anxiety, and preoccupying thoughts about the trauma.

Craig et al. (2007) proposed that *complicated grief disorder* be included in the Diagnostic and Statistical Manual of Mental Disorder (DSM IV) criteria, positing that survivors of genocide, as in the case of Servana and others from Bosnia, suffer from multiple losses. They experience the loss of family, home, a sense of belonging, a purpose in life, and mostly, a loss of hope. Their term *"complicated grief"* takes into account this sense of loss, which includes "an individual being frozen or stuck in a state of chronic mourning in which much of their mental anguish stems from their psychological protest against reality of the loss and general reluctance to make adaptations to life in the absence of a loved one." (p. 104) It is easy to see that refugees are at high risk for *complicated grief.*

War is a life-changing event. Servana's coping skills are now episodic at best. Support groups such as family, friends, and church community are not readily available as they were in Bosnia. Adding a language barrier, we can see the immense challenge before her.

> **Reflective exercise**: Violence in our lives . . .
> 1. *Do you know or have you worked with refugee populations?*
> 2. *From which country? . . . What were their experiences?*
> 3. *Think about your patient population: Have they experienced violent events?*
> 4. *If so, what resources are available for them? For you?*
> 5. *Have you ever experienced a traumatic event that affected you personally?*
> 6. *Do memories and emotions related to this event "pop up" unexpectedly?*

Who does what . . .

The federal government offers services to address those issues and provide support during resettlement. In 1980 congress passed the Refugee Act, legislation assuring equity in the treatment of refugees. The new definition no longer applies only to refugees "from communism" or certain areas of the Middle East; it now applies to all who meet the test of the United Nations Convention and Protocol on the Status of Refugees (Kennedy 1981 p. 143). It also includes a provision for those seeking asylum. The Refugee Act provides funding for programs that aid the process of adapting to a new country. According to the Office of Refugee Resettlement, 98,000 refugees enter the country each year. Unlike the immigrant, refugees sponsored by the United States government are encouraged to utilize programs such as job training, English language classes, and welfare programs. Tuition for higher education is provided as well. Case managers and social workers facilitate this process and ensure the individual is aware of available services.

Prior to entry into the United States, each person undergoes three health assessments. These are done to ensure that no communicable diseases are brought into the country. Unfortunately, little attention is paid to their mental status. Depression, anxiety, or post traumatic stress disorder (PTSD), as seen in Servana's case, can thwart attempts to learn a new language, find employment, or participate in support groups.

Process of adjustment

While we would like to think that resettlement is a process that occurs quickly, in reality it takes a long time. Isolation, as well as language, economics, and transportation, can make the adjustment process overwhelming to the refugee. The customs and cultural ways of living in the host country may add stress and may lead to feelings of helplessness, frustration, depression, and anxiety.

According to Shusta et al. (2004), there are seven stages (Figure 13-1) of adjustment for immigrants and refugees: surviving, preserving, adjusting, changing, choosing, maintaining, and expanding. This chapter focuses on the first five components. There is no set timeframe for each level, as the individual determines when to move to the next stage. As economical and educational opportunities present themselves, adjustment and acculturation occur.

Type	Status	Value
Surviving	< 5 years	Maintain one's country of origin, values, beliefs, language, customs
Preserving	> 5 years	Preserve one's cultural value & traditions; maintain community
Adjusting	2nd generation	Work hard & become assimilated
Changing	Majority in U.S.	Energy focus on changing in order to succeed
Choosing	3rd generation	Biculturalism important; be able to choose aspects of old & new cultures
Maintaining	Anticipate return	Plan to return home following work assignment (H2 Visas)
Expanding	Global	Focus on expanding globally; may speak several languages

Figure 13-1: Stages of Adjustment for Refugees & Immigrants

The chart presents a visual depiction of the stages and helps us to understand the process that these individuals have to grapple with each day. Servana is in the survival stage. Support in the form of encouragement, resources, and interest in her well-being are essential. For refugees like Servana, who have experienced violence and trauma in their country of origin, PTSD symptoms may surface. As HCPs we need to be alert to signs and symptoms of PTSD, depression, and anxiety. Other underlying issues continue to emerge as well. With each encounter HCPs have the opportunity to work collaboratively with the patient to resolve some of these issues. Interpreters, preferably bilingual/bicultural, are important during this time. Establishing a foundation of understanding and respect for the patient's experiences and dilemmas indicates that we can be counted on to be there for them during this process.

Adjusting, changing, and choosing reflect the ability and willingness to acculturate to the host country. This may not occur until the second generation, however, and is not without some conflict, especially intergenerational. Children of refugees attend school and are exposed to American cultural values and expressions, some of which may be in conflict with the parents' closely held cultural beliefs. Helping the first generation to understand the second generation may be one of the HCP's tasks. At each encounter, we continue to acknowledge the refugees' accomplishments and encourage them to pursue their dreams anew – for themselves, their families, and their communities.

Understanding the culture . . .

Cultural values, beliefs, and healthcare practices remain for a lifetime, even though one may not reside in his or her country of origin. For the Bosnian refugee, traditions and customs of the host country may be different from their own. When we incorporate their beliefs, values, and practices into the plan of care, we are sending a message that we understand and care. Listed are the cultural values of the Bosnian people pre-war.

Prewar In Bosnia
- Patriarchy
- Clearly defined roles for each family member
- Elders, especially the mother-in-law, held in high esteem
- Extended family serving to meet the needs of the family as a whole
- Communal approach of working together to provide for the needs and well-being of all members.
- In rural areas, sons were expected to remain with the father on the farm

Robertson, (Duckett 2007)

This all changed during the war. In a study by Julie Lipson (2008), the war theme is identified as "on the move" exemplified in the Bosnian mother's necessity to be constantly moving in order to protect her children – "leaving homes behind, hiding in forests, traveling from village to village just to keep ahead of the soldiers." (p. 468) Many family members, husbands, and sons were murdered during the ethnic cleansing. In July of 1995 alone over eight thousand Muslim men and boys were taken into the forest and executed. (Rohde 1997) This was denied by the government at the time, but later proven to be true.

The once familiar family life changed forever. Refugees coming to the United States, mainly displaced women and children, were challenged to maintain a family unit. Following a husband's death, a widow is to "live in grief forever" and is not permitted to marry again. Reliance on extended community is vital to survival.

As HCPs we are called to be part of that process in assisting the refugees in rebuilding their lives. It can begin by acknowledging their loss of place and family and the increased stress produced by caring for themselves and their children in a foreign country. As we listen to their stories, we can assist them in identifying needs and finding resources and we can teach them how to navigate through the healthcare system. Servana's educational level and skills can translate to job opportunities here. Resources for all refugees must include counseling, support groups, language classes, and job training opportunities.

Communication

The Bosnian language spoken is similar to the Serbo-Croatian dialect. Religion, gender, and political or social backgrounds may influence the style of communication. Tone of voice is respectful and conversation is direct and sincere and centers on the subject at hand. Since Yugoslavia was "westernized" prior to the war, its people adopted much of the western style, including direct eye contact, a firm hand shake, and even an embrace. They are generally friendly and open, and losing one's temper is thought to be impolite. It is also important to avoid conflict.

For the refugee who speaks no English, there may be some distrust toward an interpreter (based on previous experiences). Given the trauma this person may have experienced during the war, a linguistically, culturally, and socially competent interpreter is essential. It is helpful for the HCP to meet with the interpreter prior to the session to establish clear expectations and guidelines. Mental health issues may be difficult for the patient to discuss as it causes him or her to relive traumatic events. It may take several encounters, in fact, before that discussion can take place, especially since mental illness may have a negative stigma. Some Bosnian refugees are afraid of deportation if mental health issues were to be discovered.

Expectations of health . . . and care

Bosnian refugees, like others who come to this country, can be highly educated professionals or they may be from rural areas of the country. Caution must be taken not to stereotype refugees by speaking down to them as if they were uneducated and unwilling to participate fully in their care. At home Bosnians were used to a state-run health system, similar in many ways to the healthcare in the United States. An individual was seen at a local clinic or could just drop in, as appointments were not necessary. Physician home visits were available as well. According to Bosnian refugee participants in a study by Lipson et al. (2008), there was usually a strong relationship between the patient and the physician and that "the universal system of health care in Yugoslavia was a source of pride." Part of a good resettlement program includes access to refugee clinics that have on-site interpreters. Insurance is provided through the government-run healthcare program.

Other that the use of herbal remedies in the case of minor illness, there is very little specific information about the healthcare practices of the non-Muslim Bosnian. The American values of self-reliance, independence, and empowerment to "do for yourself" may not be consistent with the Bosnian value placed on communal existence and reliance on extended family. Facilitating networking for Bosnian refugees may improve quality of life and assure a support system that is readily accessible.

Reflective exercise: Quality of life . . .
1. *What support groups are available for the refugees in your area?*
2. *Are case managers and social workers available?*
3. *Does your cultural health assessment tool address the needs of persons with refugee status?*
4. *Does the assessment include questions about mental status?*

When elderly cannot care for themselves . . .

Nursing homes are not an option in Bosnian culture; family and/or close friends are responsible for the care of the elderly. It is considered disrespectful in the eyes of many Bosnians for a family to turn its back on providing care for its elders. "It is your moral obligation to take care of your parents, poor and rich alike," stated Lydia Hamzic, a Bosnian woman who teaches ESL (English as a Second Language) in Utica, New York. "People would spit on you if they knew you placed your parents in a home." Further, a nursing home would be especially detrimental to the wellbeing of an aged Bosnian in America because most do not know the language. Lydia said, "No elderly person would last more than a couple of months in a nursing home, s/he would die of a broken heart." However, Bosnians welcome home healthcare as a vehicle for providing information about services for the elderly, and additional resources in the community may be helpful to the patient and family as well.

*   *   *   *

Bosnians and many other refugees have been traumatized in their country of origin. Relocating to a host country, while helping to dispel fears of torture, rape, or death, may add a new layer of stress. Coping on a daily basis with this newness is overwhelming, and unfortunately it adds to the physical and mental health issues of the refugee. Our job as HCPs is to be aware, to ask questions gently, to encourage family participation, and mostly to be the resource that enables the person to adjust to this new way of living in the larger world.

Culture Care Modes & Actinos
Bosnian Refugee – PTSD

Preservation/Maintenance
- Family support
- Communication style

Accommodation/Negotiation
- Educational opportunities
- Interpreters ~ bilingual/bicultural

Repatterning/Restructuring
- Addressing PTSD with options such as biofeedback, medication, and behavioral therapy

Resources

Allotey, P., Manderson, L., Nikles, J., Reidpath, D., Sauvarin, J. (2008). Cultural Divrsity: Bosnian Muslims. University of Queensland. Retrieved on November 1, 2009, from http://qhin.health.qid, gov.au/hssb/hou/hom.html

Corvo, K., Peterson, J. (2005). Post-traumatic stress symptoms, language, acquisition and self sufficiency. *Journal of Social Work.* (5)2, 205-219.

Craig, C. D., Sossou, M. A., Schnak, M., Essex, H. (2008). Complicated grief and its relationship to mental health and well-being among Bosnian refugees after resettlement in the United States: Implications for practice, policy and research. *Traumatology.* (14)4, 103-115.

DeSantis, L. (1997). Building health communities with immigrants and refugees. *Journal of Transcultural Nursing.* (9)1, 20-29.

Douglas, M. (1999). "Ethnic cleansing": The ultimate tragedy of intolerance. *Journal of Transcultural Nursing.* (10)2, 93.

Hamzic, E. St. Elizabeth Medical Center. Cultural Diversity: Bosnians. Retrieved July 1, 2009 from http://www.stemc.org/about_stemc/cultural_diversity/bosnians

Husain, S. A., Allwood, M. A., Bell, D. J. (2008). The relationship between PTSD symptoms and attention problems in children exposed to the Bosnian War. *Journal of Educational and Behavorial Disorders.* (16)1, 52-62.

Kennedy, E. (1981). Refugee Act of 1980. International Migration Review. (15) 1/2, p. 141-156.

Lipson, J. G., Weinstein, H. M., Gladstone, E. A., Sarnoff, R. H. (2003). Bosnian and Soviet refugees' experiences with health care. *Western Journal of Nursing Research.* (25)7, 854-871.

Purnell, L. (2009). People of Bosnian Heritage. *Guide to Culturally Competent Health Care.* (2nd Ed.). Philadelphia PA: F.A. Davis.

Robertson, C. L., Duckett, L. D. (2007). Mothering during war and postwar in Bosnia. *Journal of Family Nursing.* (13)4, 461-483.

Rohlof, H., Knipscheer, J. W., Kleber, R. J. (2009). Use of the cultural formulation with refugees. *Transcultural Psychiatry.* (46)3, 487-505.

Simpson, J. L., Carter, K. (2008). Muslim women's experiences with health care providers in a rural area of the United States. *Journal of Transcultural Nursing.* (19)1, 16-23.

Shusta, R. M., Levine, D. R., Wong, H. Z., Olson, A. T., Harris, P. R. (2008). *Multicultural Law Enforcement: Strategies for Peacekeeping in a Diverse Society*. (4th Ed.) New Jersey: Pearson, Prentice Hall.

Tellep, T. L., Morakath, C., Murphy, S., Cureton, V. J. (2001). Great suffering, great compassion: A transcultural opportunity for school nurses caring for Cambodian refugee children. *Journal of Transcultural Nursing*. (12)4, 261-274.

Standing Tall and Proud
(Native American)

14

Prior to the 1930s there was only one documented case of diabetes in the Southwest tribes. They now have one of the highest rates in the world (Knowler, Bennett, Hamman & Miller 1978).

What happened? A domino effect of dramatic changes in the tribes' lifestyle after the U.S. Government constructed dams on the Gila River.

First, diverting the water dried up the local hunting, fishing, and farming opportunities, causing their physically demanding regime to give way to more sedentary habits.

That was followed by the commodity food program, an attempt by the federal government to offset these losses. The Indians' traditionally low-fat, low-sugar diet was replaced with shipments of foods high in carbohydrates, including flour, white bread, lard, canned meat, peanut butter, and cheese.

The PBS film (2008), Unnatural Causes: Is Inequality Making Us Sick, documents the link between the diversion of water in the Gila river to the current day diabetes crisis in the Pima Indians.

* * * *

Standing Tall and Proud

Billy remembers going hungry. He remembers days when the deer weren't easy to come by, when even squirrels seemed out of reach up in the tree. He never was much of a hunter, but he remembers the stories his grandfather told him when they'd hang out together by Mount Shasta, the holy mountain. His grandfather was a great hunter and provider. Billy also remembers, as he grew to manhood,

165

the tears of his father. It is an awful thing not to be able to provide for one's family. After the white people came and moved the Littlejohns and their clan away from the Lake, times were hard. Even the sweat lodge could not steam away the pain.

Billy can still feel that twang in his stomach, kind of like the ones made by those guitar riffs that reach him and his nephews out here on the rez on that country station KBOY. Not so acute now, though. Ever since the government saw fit to recognize some of the damage done to his people, there's been enough food – lots of peanut butter and cheese, what with all the subsidies. The Littlejohns have always hated hand-outs, but it has been good not to feel that twang. And Billy has grown to love PB and J's and American cheese.

Mary Sue and Elena will arrive soon. They're government too, but nice enough, kind of like peanut butter instead of venison.

The heat that penetrates his porch roof would be too much of a gift without the oak that shades it. Billy smiles as he thinks of his blessings: sunshine, tobacco, shelter, solitude, what family he has left. Even though his parents and his sister Winnie have passed on, they are very present in his mind. He wonders how they are, whether they have gone to a place beyond this world or whether they have become part of it, part of the stones and the river and the earth itself. As the nurse and the social worker pull up in their Acura, he readies himself for more sermons on the future of his body. Rising and tipping his hat, Billy stands as tall as is now possible, what with the diabetes.

"Well hello, Mr. Littlejohn. Have you taken our words to heart? Are you cutting back on those 'roll-your-owns'?" Elena is always concerned about his health first, but that's her job. She worries that Billy will be out here under his tree and unable to see, that his leg might need amputation, especially if he keeps on with the cigarettes. At least he doesn't drink. She thinks Billy doesn't realize how lucky he is to be part of this great nation. Her Hungarian relatives were all killed in one of those freedom fights back in '56.

Mary Sue focuses on where he will live. Certainly a shack in the woods, even if it's part of the reservation, won't do in a year or two. "I've found real nice places for some of your people in town, Billy. New linoleum. Air-conditioning. Shag carpets."

Watching as the two women step briskly up the porch stairs, Billy steps back a bit, extending his hand tentatively. He keeps standing, waiting for them to sit first. "Sure hope they don't grab and shake like the last time," he's thinking. He looks down. Billy can hear the creek down the hill, not the rapid springtime flow, but still moving along. Kind of like me. He can hear a jay near the top of the madrone too, just one, but one but you can always hear jays. Sure are a pretty blue.

Elena and Mary Sue fidget in the silence; no creek, no joys, just someone who needs to focus on his options for the next few years. Elena gets out her cuff to take

Billy's pressure. That'll be something to do and they require one at the clinic of course, even though it's not the pressure but the blood sugar that's the problem. He just doesn't seem to think about anything but sitting on this old porch. And they have six other Indians to check in on while they're out here. All six seem to be off in a dream world too.

After a series of the usual questions about Billy's sleep, difficulty breathing, dizziness, numbness, change in vision, any unusual skin ulceration, each answered monosyllabically and noted in Elena's book, she proceeds to the corroborative tests. It's pretty hard to do a good physical on a clothed man but she manages; with all the movies about naked braves riding into battle, Billy's modesty still surprises her. According to him, he's healthy as his pinto mare. According to the vision and skin reactivity tests Elena employs, he has a couple of years until he can't see or feel his right leg below his knee. Same old, same old. While Mary Sue makes a circuit of the house taking her own notes for the agency, Elena sighs and packs her paraphernalia back into its bag. Billy sighs too as he realizes that his physical is over.

"If only they'd leave me in peace," he muses. Elena and Mary Sue, frustrated and perspiring more that they'd like, hurry back to the Acura to turn on the AC.

"If only he'd consider his future," Mary Sue signs as she pulls away down the dirt road. "Sometimes I just about give up on these Indians," Elena concurs.

* * * *

There are more than 500 federally recognized Native American tribes in the United States. Each is a unique community with traditions, culture, beliefs, and language. In our scenario both Elena and Mary Sue referred to Mr. Littlejohn as "Indian." What is the respectful way to address a person: American Indian, Native American, or Indian? The United States Census Bureau uses the term American Indian. What are the appropriate and respectful terms? Five Native American nurse scholars, each with different tribal affiliation, were asked to respond to that question:

"I use Native American and American Indian interchangeably." "I was taught that I am a Cherokee first, then an Indian, and then a U.S. citizen." Struthers, Lauderdale, Nichols, Tom-Orme & Stickland 2003 p.194

As HCPs we can begin the conversation with our patients by simply asking how they wish to be addressed. Defining the word "health" from the patients' perspective should be next on the agenda.

Wellness Is . . .

Bringing Wellness Home, a conference sponsored by the Pomo Indian tribe of Northern California, began with a dance and incantation that acknowledged the four directions, north, south, east and west. Billy Rogers, the keynote speaker and Director of the Native Wellness Institute in Norman, Oklahoma, provided us with a visual depiction of Wellness Is . . . as shown in Figure 14-1. The four intersecting circles (wheels) – spiritual, emotional, physical, and mental – influence and are affected by each other. They are integral in maintaining health in one's life. Wellness, as Billy Rogers notes, is found when there is balance and harmony within each component.

The cultural beliefs, values, and health practices found in the Native American population are in alignment with Billy Rogers' "Wellness Is. . ." model. The circular nature of life promotes balance in relationships and in the environment. Harmony comes also with respect for elders and tribal leadership.

Native American Cultural Beliefs & Values

1. Harmony
2. Respect for the environment
3. Pride in traditions and rituals
4. Folk healers and practices
5. Circular nature of life
6. Authority of leaders
7. Respect for elders and their wisdom
8. Children are highly valued and are the future

<u>Reflective exercise</u>: **Cultural Beliefs and Values**
1. *In what ways are your values different from those listed?*
2. *Where do you find common ground?*
3. *In what ways do you find/establish balance in your life?*

Family and Kinship

Kinship structure varies from culture to culture. Some nations are patriarchal and others matriarchal. Status or importance comes with age and experience, not with education or economic status. Collaboration and sharing of resources are essential to the well-being of the family and community. Extended family, highly valued in the Native American culture, ensures support and assistance especially during times of illness, disability, and death. This collectivistic approach highlights the group and not the individual. Family and tribal associations are highly valued and appreciated. For those of us in the healthcare setting, this may translate into several family members being present during a clinical appointment or during hospitalization.

WELLNESS IS...

- A holistic model to help guide us along a path of BALANCE.
- An integrated approach in the way people live their lives. There are four directions to wellness: *physical, mental, emotional*, and *spiritual*.
- Dependent on the individual's potential for personal growth, it is being "all you can be".
- Most importantly, native wellness embraces the teachings of the old ways – living life in a circle.

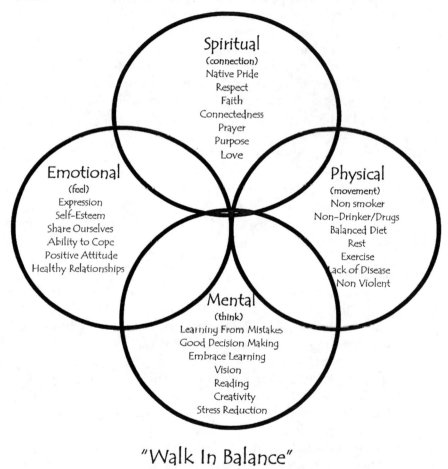

Spiritual
(connection)
Native Pride
Respect
Faith
Connectedness
Prayer
Purpose
Love

Emotional
(feel)
Expression
Self-Esteem
Share Ourselves
Ability to Cope
Positive Attitude
Healthy Relationships

Physical
(movement)
Non smoker
Non-Drinker/Drugs
Balanced Diet
Rest
Exercise
Lack of Disease
Non Violent

Mental
(think)
Learning From Mistakes
Good Decision Making
Embrace Learning
Vision
Reading
Creativity
Stress Reduction

"Walk In Balance"

Billy Rogers
Native Wellness Institute
Norman, Oklahoma
June 2002

Figure 14-2: Wellness Is . . .
Billy Rodgers, Native Wellness Institute, Norman, Oklahoma;Used with permission.

The role of father and mother continue to evolve secondary to economic and social shifts in society. The traditional role of the mother caring for the home and children while the father works outside the home is changing due to financial instability. Unfortunately this may cause families to move away from the security and support of the extended family. Children are highly valued members of the family. They are taught at an early age to respect their elders and take pride in tribal traditions. While autonomy and independence are encouraged, the child knows that consequences are possible and that decisions can affect the family and the community. Children are encouraged by their parents and extended family to live and learn by their decisions (Giger & Davidhizar, 2008 p. 282). Elders are respected and revered members of the family and community. They are the keepers of the wisdom and are responsible to pass knowledge on to the next generation.

While decision making is thought to be an autonomous activity and no one person speaks for another, a family member may speak for the individual if he or she is unable, due to illness

Reflective excersize: American Indian Family
1. *How is your family different?*
2. *As a child, were you given independence and autonomy?*
3. *Does extended family accompany you to appointments?*
4. *How were decisions made in your family? . . . Is that the same today?*
5. *Where do you find common ground?*

Communication

Depending on the source, there are between 150 to 200 indigenous languages spoken. On a recent trip to the southwest, the conversation in the local cafe was in Navajo. While some of the elderly continue to speak in their native tongue, many tribes are encouraging their younger members to "learn the language before it is lost forever."

The Native American style of communication may use metaphors and anecdotes to discuss a situation. This provides clarification through the use of examples. Speech is usually tonal and pitch plays a significant role in the meaning. Loud expressions may be seen as aggressive and rude. While there may be long pauses during the conversation, the HCP is encouraged to wait, especially when allowing an elder to respond. Interest is shown through silence. Not allowing time may actually result in an incorrect response or cause the patient to offer no response. The following is a handout, Learning to Listen (Figure 14-2), received during the Pomo Wellness conference. While it is directed at native youth, it can be an example for the HCP to use in the every day.

Respectful communication is demonstrated by avoiding eye contact or using it sparingly. Pointing a finger may be considered an insult, thus the patient may indicate direction by shifting their lips toward the desired direction instead of pointing (Coutu-Wakulczyk 2004 et al. p 281). Touch is extended to those who are known to the patient. In many tribes, touch is a common practice, especially in traditional healing ceremonies. As an outsider, the HCP should establish a relationship with the patient before touch is considered acceptable. A light handshake is acceptable.

According to Rachel Spector in her book Cultural Diversity in Health and Wellness, note taking is taboo. Native American history has been passed through generations by means of storytelling. Native Americans are sensitive about note taking when they are speaking. When taking a history or interviewing, it may be preferable to use memory skills rather than to record notes. The more conversational approach may encourage greater openness between the patient and the provider (2009, p. 226).

Time and Space

Time orientation focuses on personal and seasonal rhythms. Events may not have a defined time but rather begin when the group gathers. For the Native American, present day orientation values being in harmony with people and nature. Past orientation, valued as well, correlates with the cultural value of oral history, respect for tradition, elders, and ancestors. The focus of future orientation is children and education.

The HCP should focus on the present moment and present needs. When asking a question that requires more than a yes or no answer, allow time for the patient to respond. Treatment plans, developed in collaboration with the patient, focus on "here and now" goals. For example, review the patient's food intake from that day and obtain a blood sugar. This is especially helpful if the patient feels well and does not see the need to take his or her medicine. The visual of both the food diary and the blood sugar level will provide a better understanding and a better health outcome.

Listening	Body Language
• Use responses like "I see" & "umm"	• Sit down when talking
• Use reflective question	• Avoid too much eye contact
• It's OK to have extended "pause" time	• Keep arms unfolded
• Be patient and don't interrupt	• Affirm with head nods

Figure 14-2: Learning to Listen
Native Wellness Institute (2002). Used with permission

171

<u>Reflective exercise</u>: Communication and Time
1. *How is your communication style the same or different?*
2. *How comfortable are you with long periods of silence?*
3. *How would you modify your approach?*
4. *In what ways could you incorporate present day orientation into the plan of care?*

Healing beliefs ~ Family, Community, and Expectations

In the opening scene of the movie Whale Rider, a group of Maori are gathered around the hospital bed of a young woman who is dying. Consistent with traditional values, the extended family is present, and the singers and drummers provide support for the journey to the next world. In many hospital settings across the United States, similar scenes are taking place. Realizing the importance of family and end-of-life concerns, many hospitals now provide a venue in which these ceremonies can take place.

This section began with a hospital scene from Whale Rider to illustrate the significance of people's cultural beliefs and practices, and the weight placed on healing beliefs and practices. For the American Indian, health and well-being are not only in direct relationship to the physical body, but also to family, environment, spiritual forces, and community. Illness occurs when there is an imbalance. The role of the sick person is to be quiet and stoic. Healing comes from their traditional holistic and wellness approach in combination with western medicine.

Native healers may be called medicine men or women, and in the Navajo tradition may serve different roles such as diagnostician, singer, or herbalist. As implied, the diagnostician diagnoses the cause of the disharmony, the singers perform and direct healing ceremonies, and the herbalist diagnoses and identifies herbs that promote healing. Working collaboratively, healers and HCPs can share information and discuss healing modes and practices. This demonstrates to the patients the acceptance of and respect for their beliefs and healthcare practices.

<u>Reflective exercise</u>: Healing practices and relationships
1. *In what ways are healers invited to participate in the care of your patient?*
2. *Is staff knowledgeable about the cultural health beliefs and practices of the population?*
3. *In what ways do your health beliefs and practices match your patient population?*
4. *Who are the healers?*
5. *How would you modify your approach, given this information?*

Using Storytelling with Education

Mr. Littlejohn talks about the value of balance and rhythm in his life. A visual depiction of that balance is seen in the Medicine Wheel (Figure 14-1), a symbol of wholeness. This model shared by Ann Dapice (2006) was developed by staff at a mental health facility. Similar to the Balance of the Four Humors with elements of season, temperature, moisture, body fluids, and personality found in Chapter 9, the Medicine Wheel displays similar components. Each section highlights a direction, aspect of health, color, animal, and medicine and all must be in balance to ensure health and wellness of the individual.

Direction—North
Aspect—Spiritual
Color—White
Animal—White Buffalo
Medicine—Sweetgrass

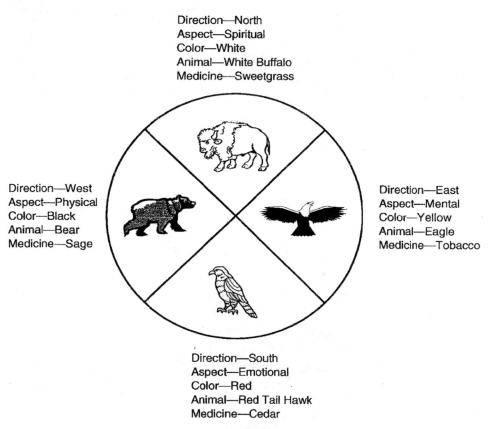

Direction—West
Aspect—Physical
Color—Black
Animal—Bear
Medicine—Sage

Direction—East
Aspect—Mental
Color—Yellow
Animal—Eagle
Medicine—Tobacco

Direction—South
Aspect—Emotional
Color—Red
Animal—Red Tail Hawk
Medicine—Cedar

Figure 14-3: Medicine Wheel
Source: Used with permission; Ann N. Dapice TCNJ 2006 17 p. 25

Given this information, Elena and Mary Sue might inquire how Billy Littlejohn views his illness and treatment options. What does he think he needs to get better? Does he use folk practices such as a sweat lodge or medicinal herbs? A final question for Elena and Mary Sue: Do our educational materials reflect Billy's culture?

"Diabetes Prevention in Indian Country: Developing Nutritional Models to Tell the Story of Food-System Change" (2006), written by Kibbe Conti, a Certified Diabetic Educator, is an excellent article. She posits that when cultural beliefs, values, and health practices are integrated into the diabetic educational material, results are better than good, they are great! She combines the values of respect for tradition and storytelling, along with the symbol of the Medicine Wheel, to convey the message. The initial model tells the story of the dietary habits prior to the initiation of the dams and relocation, and each succeeding model from that time frame to the present shows changes in nutritional habits. The purpose is to bring about an awareness using narrative and imagery. The educational material used as a "talking tool" can be modified to fit with any patient population.

In her article she highlights the diabetic teaching tool developed by the Mandan/Hidatsa/Arikara Nations of North Dakota. Utilizing the medicine wheel, they provide both visual and narrative elements to demonstrate the dietary and activity changes that have taken place over the past one hundred plus years. Notice the changes as you read about each era. Each wheel depicts a specific era, and through a visual narrative shows changes in dietary habits. From pre-dam status to the effects of the federal food commodity program in the 1940s to current day healthy food choices, the patient can see the effect of inadequate nutrition over time.

Traditional Food Pattern Pre-1880s
*Hunting and fishing and farming
*Fresh foods and pure water
*Active lifestyle

Loss of the Bottomlands – Loss of Food Traditions (Diabetes emerges)
*Loss of farming, hunting & fishing
*Loss of fresh and available water
*Reliance on food commoditities
*Change in activity

Eating out of Balance – Mid-1950s
* Processed foods
*Sweetened drinks
*Sedentary lifestyle

Restoring Balance with Healthier Choices
*Medicine wheel format instead of pyramid chart
*Healthy food selection options
*Increase activity

Storytelling, a method used in health education, is congruent with the oral tradition found in the Native American population. The storyteller uses examples of history, food intake, and consequences of dietary choices to assist the patient in identifying cultural values that connect with tribal traditions. These stories provide an opportunity for the listener/patient to interpret and draw conclusions. If done within a family, a group, or in a tribal community setting, this dialogue promotes and reinforces cultural values, beliefs, and healthcare practices. It was noted by the author that Native American patients using the tool found it easier to understand than the food pyramid.

Reflective exercise: Educational material for diabetic patients
1. *Who are your patients?*
2. *Is your educational material culturally balanced?*
3. *With your patient population, what educational format is most successful in achieving results?*
4. *What changes might you make?*
5. *Who needs to be part of that process . . . educators, patients, community leaders?*

*   *   *   *

Billy Littlejohn's cultural beliefs, values and healthcare practices, passed down from generation to generation, are essential components in determining outcomes. The knowledge and motivation by the HCP to incorporate those health practices into the plan of care not only helps to assure rapport and respect, but also is a portent of positive health outcomes. The knowledge and motivation by the HCP to incorporate those health practices into the plan of care helps to assure rapport and respect for the patient. As Alice Dupine stated, "the clients found the traditional tools more effective than the dietary pyramid." How can you incorporate this information into your approach when dealing with your clients?

Culture Care Modes & Actions
Native American – Diabetes

Preservation/Maintenance
- Respect for the elderly and those in authority
- Family support
- Tradition and history

Accommodation/Negotiation
- Inclusion of family in educational setting
- Folk practices
- Balance of hot and cold

Repatterning/Restructuring
- Diet ~ healthy choices
- Exercise

Resources

Abbott, P. D., Short, E., Dodson, S., Garcia, C., Perkins, J., Wyant, S. (2002). Improving your cultural awareness with culture clues. *Nurse Practitioner.* 27(2), 44-51.

Andrews, M. M., Boyle, J. S. (2008). *Transcultural concepts in nursing care*. (5th Ed.).New York: Lippincott Williams & Wilkins.

Campinha-Bacote, J. (2002). Readings & resources in transcultural health care and mental health. (13th Ed.).

Conti, K. M. (2006). Diabetes prevention in Indian country: Developing nutrition models to tell the story of food-system change. *Journal of Transcultural Nursing.* (17)3, 234-245.

Dapice, A. N. (2006). The Medicine Wheel. *Journal of Transcultural Nursing.* (17)3, 251-260.

De Vera, N. (2003). Perspectives on healing foot ulcers by Yaquis with diabetes. *Journal of Transcultural Nursing.* (14)1, 39-47.

Edgerly, C. C., Laing, S. S., Day, A. G., Blackinton, P. M., Pingatore, N. L., Haverkate, R. T., Heany, J. F. (2009). Steps to a healthier Anishinaabe, Micigan: Strategies for Implementing health promotion programs in multiple American Indian communities. *Health Promotion Practice.* (10)2, 109S-117S.

Galanti, G. A. (2004). Caring for patients from different cultures. (4th Ed.) University of Pennsylvania Press: Philadelphia, PA.

Hanley, C. E. (2008). Navajos. In Giger, J. N., Davidhizar, R. E. (Eds). Transcultural Nursing: Assessment and Intervention. (5th Ed.). St Louis, MO: Mosby/Elsevier.

Hodge, F. S., Pasqua, B. A., Marquez, C. A., Cantrell, B. G. (2001). Utilizing traditional storytelling to promote wellness in American Indian communities. *Journal of Transcultural Nursing.* 13(1), 6-11.

Hodgins, O., Hodgins, D. (2008). Navajo Indians. In Purnell, L. D., Paulanka, B. J. (Eds) Transcultural Health Care: A Culturally Competent Approach. (3rd Ed.). Philadelphia, PA: F. A. Davis Company.

Holkup, P. A. (2002). Big changes in the Indian Health Service: Are nurses aware? *Journal of Transcultural Nursing.* (13)1, 47-53.

Leininger, M. M., McFarland, M. R. (2002). Transcultural nursing: Concepts, theories, research and practice. (3rd Ed.). New York: McGraw-Hill.

Palacios, J., Butterfly, R., Strickland, C.J. (2005). American Indians. In Lipson, J. G., Dibble, S. L., (Eds.) Culture & Clinical Care. San Francisco CA: UCSF Nursing Press.

Sutton, C. T., Broken Nose, M. A. (2005). American Indian Families: An Overview. In McGoldrick, M.M., Giordano, J., Garcia-Preto, N. (Eds) *Ethnicity & Family Therapy*. (3rd Ed). New York: Guilford Press

Draining My Life Source . . .
Doesn't Anyone Care?
(Hmong)

15

"Where is my wife?" Seng Pao speaks very softly into his pillow, avoiding the stares of the nurses who still surround him. He is speaking in his own dialect, not English, the stress of his situation having sent him back to Laos and earlier times.

Despite his seventy-three years, he struggles to reach the tube in his nose. Those nurses put it there when Kia Pa brought him here to St. Mary's emergency this morning. But the tube is sucking out his life blood.

"Where is my wife?" Seng Pao whispers again.

At home in Laos he would be regarded as an elder, would be left his dignity; here in the States his opinion seems to be irrelevant. Here his wife even earns more money than he does. He can't find a job, after all the intelligence he gathered for the CIA in the 60s.

That's why Seng ended up here at the emergency room. Usually he just relied on his family's animal spirits to make his stomach pain go away. This morning, though, it felt as if a knife had been thrust right into his middle.

"At least I have my ankle bracelet to keep my soul inside," he thinks.

He moves his left leg laboriously on top of where the bracelet is supposed to sit, but he can not feel it under the sheets.

"They couldn't have taken it off, could they?"

Seng presumes that there are spirits watching over him here in St. Mary's too. The crucifix on the wall doesn't have any relevance in his life, but he can see the leaves of a yellow tree fluttering in the wind outside. That is a good sign. Modesto has no mountains, but it does have trees.

Seng is not an angry man. His people, the Hmong, do not get angry. But his life blood is leaving him through the tube. He will have to rely on his ancestors and his family still living for comfort and protection.

"If only they could be with me in my distress," he reflects.

"All comfortable now?" the short blond nurse asks. "Can you hear me?"

179

she shouts, touching him on the shoulder as her face nears his ear. "Ok in there?"
"Yes," he cringes.
Seng's stomach throbs, his ankle bracelet is gone, his very life is being sucked
out of his body. And family, the center of his world so far from his clan, is being
excluded from his space here behind the curtain.

This vignette is based on an actual case that occurred in the emergency room at a local hospital. Sharon Johnson chronicles the event in her article, "Hmong Health Beliefs and Experiences in the Western Health Care System" (2002). She shares information about the Hmong culture that is vital for all to know. As HCPs we are challenged each time we encounter a patient or colleague whose cultural beliefs, values, and healthcare practices are different from our own. However, it is through these experiences and sharing of stories that we learn. We tuck away those bits of information and use them in future encounters. What do you know about the Hmong culture?

It begins with . . . their story

Living in China, the Hmong were always the brunt of derogatory remarks and abusive treatment by the Chinese. Yet they stood firm as a group, as a clan, and never assimilated to the Chinese culture. To avoid continued persecution by the Chinese, they migrated to Indochina, now known as Laos, Cambodia, and Vietnam in the 1800s. Later that century, the French occupied Indochina causing several revolts by the Hmong. In 1920 the French granted the mountain area of Laos to the Hmong, which minimized contact with those living in the lowlands.

In 1954, the Geneva Accord recognized three independent countries: Vietnam, Cambodia, and Laos. Vietnam was partitioned into the North (USSR) and South (U.S.). Laos was considered a neutral country. At the Geneva Conference in 1961, it was agreed that no foreign troops or military personnel were to be sent into that region. However, because of the Hmong's knowledge of the region and their disdain for the communist government, they were recruited as advisors by the CIA (Central Intelligence Agency) to help cut the military supply line between North and South Vietnam. Many were killed in this conflict, and the results were devastating for their families left behind. Post war, villages were unable to sustain the population due to the labor shortage. In addition, due to their alliance with the Americans, the Hmong faced certain torture and death at the hands of the new government.

Survival meant migration. The many years spent at refugee camps in Thailand strengthened their values of clan loyalty and solidarity. Once in the U.S., anticipated eligibility for veterans' benefits (because of their work with the CIA) was not forthcoming, thus requiring application for public assistance. The stigma of taking something for nothing followed them wherever they lived in the United States. Today the the Hmong people reside primarily in California, with others in Minnesota, Wisconsin, North Carolina, and Colorado. Adherence to traditional cultural values has grown stronger as their world changed forever.

Hmong Cultural Values & Beliefs

The foundation . . . cultural beliefs and traditions
- Clan and family loyalty
- Hierarchy and patriarchy
- Animism and power of the spirit world
- Independent group spirit
- Ancestor worship

Solidarity as a group is the foundation of their belief. Their fierce independent spirit avoids assimilation as demonstrated during occupation by the French or now when living in the United States. The eighteen clans currently in the United States provide security and stability for families. Families are hierarchal and patriarchal. The male ranks higher than the female, and the elderly over the youth. It is said that "ten young men equal one old man," which gives us a sense of the significance of an elderly male such as Seng Pao. Loyalty extends beyond death, as ancestor worship affords protection for the family, especially in times of serious illness.

Family Hierarchy and Loyalty

In *The Spirit Catches You and You Fall Down* (1996), a story about a Hmong family living in the central valley of California, author Anne Fadiman shares the Hmong belief that "to be with a family is to be happy, to be without is to be lost."

The husband is considered the head of the household and makes the family decisions about finances, relationships, and education. In the Hmong beliefs, a man can have more that one wife. This is a common practice in their homeland and, while unlawful in the United States, it continues to be practiced. An article in the *Milwaukee Journal* (2006) tells the story about a young Hmong woman who, after arriving in the United States with her family, tells of her father taking an additional wife and bringing her home to live with his current family. Though resentful and uncomfortable with the situation, she accepts this as part of her Hmong culture.

Women's role is primarily that of caregiver and nurturer. However, immigration brought about unanticipated changes: relocation to urban areas, clan members living thousands of miles apart; and high unemployment for men. Women, who previously worked inside the home and provided for the family, now work outside the home, sometimes making more money than their husbands. The change in roles and responsibilities may increase tension, thus affecting health.

Children belong to their father's clan. They are taught to honor the beliefs and practices of the Hmong culture, particularly to respect those in authority. Transition to a new life in the United States has been difficult for the children as well. As a result of attending school in the United States and speaking English, they are called on to translate for their parents and elders. It puts them in a position of power that is not in keeping with the Hmong hierarchical structure. They live in two different worlds: school and home. In the school environment, they are encouraged to speak up and "think for themselves," while at home they are expected to be reserved and give deference to their parents and the elderly. Different expectations can be frustrating. However, a recent report shared that the more aligned a Hmong college student is with his or her ethnicity, the better he or she does academically.

The elderly are held in high esteem. They are expected to contribute to the family through sharing their wisdom and caring for grandchildren. Interestingly, even after death they are considered part of the family, because their spirits continue to protect and guide family members.

Decision making is in the hands of the clan leader, and he must be consulted prior to any agreement for significant health services. Seng Pao and family may wait for the clan leader to arrive before agreeing to a procedure or surgery. It could take days. And the family will wait. Reflecting on Seng Pao's situation, it is vital that we as HCPs understand the importance and significance of the clan leader and the family.

Communication

Hmong people are steeped in the oral tradition. First written down in the 1950s by a missionary, the Hmong language uses multiple words to describe a situation or condition, where one word in the English language may suffice. Transitioning from a primarily oral language culture to one that requires proficiency in reading, writing, and speaking can be a daunting task for the Hmong patient. Translation is not literally word for word, and Western medical terms may not translate into the Hmong language.

Translation services in the Hmong dialect are limited or nonexistent in many healthcare settings. When unfamiliar with another's language, there is a tendency to speak louder to ensure understanding. This is the case with Seng Pao when the nurse says loudly to Seng Pao, "can you hear me?" "okay in there?" The translation process may be lengthy. Allowing more time shows respect for the patient. What are some other ways to show respect to Seng Pao? Anne Fadiman offers some suggestions.

Suggestions for female HCPs when meeting with Hmong men:
- Don't raise your voice
- Take off your shoes
- Don't offer to shake hands
    - ☐ If a man offers . . . indicate your lower status
    - ☐ Place left hand under your right wrist in order to support the weight of his honored and important hand
- Walk behind and to the left of Hmong leader
- Use older male interpreter to compensate for your lack of status
- Never say no to an offer of food

Fadiman, Anne (1996 p.93)

Respect for elderly and those in authority includes minimal eye contact and avoidance of conflict. Polite listening and nodding of the head by the patient while verbally saying "yes" may really mean "no." Or it may mean "I don't understand." These responses may be used to maintain dignity and save face. Touch is also to be avoided. Always ask permission first before touching.

Tone of voice for the Hmong patient is usually soft. The speed of the conversation may seem fast due to the monosyllabic words used to convey the message. The patient may appear stoic and display minimal emotion, though nonverbal cues may convey another meaning. Allowing time and not rushing the appointment provides an opportunity to build rapport and trust.

The cycle of time . . .

In the Hmong way of life farming in the hill country of Laos, time was relative to cycles of the seasons of planting and harvesting. The day began with the first cock crow, followed by the second cock crow, the time the sun inclined, the time shadows covered the valley, the pig feeding time, and ended with full darkness (Fadiman, 1996). Transition to an urban way of life in the United States with emphasis on punctuality and future planning is not synonymous with the old ways where more attention is given to the present moment. The result may mean that the Hmong patient may not arrive at the specified time for an appointment. When the HCP's time orientation and patients are not aligned, misunderstanding and conflict can ensue. Flexibility is not always an option for the HCP, but adaptation may bring about mutual respect.

Health beliefs

The Hmong hold an animistic belief that all things in nature – plants, winds, and hills – have a soul. Taoism, a Chinese philosophy incorporating the underlying principles of Yin and Yang, are also included in these beliefs. Health and wellbeing are directly related to balance and harmony in one's life. Illness is an imbalance in the natural world, such as vulnerability to the elements (wind and cold air), exposure to chemicals, or consumption of spoiled food or tainted water. Treatment is found in the concept of Yin and Yang. Health is restored through such methods as cupping (removing wind from the body), coining, massaging, pinching (to draw out the noxious wind), and ingesting herbal teas.

Not having a complete understanding of the anatomy of the the body, the Hmong believe there is a finite amount of blood within the body. Drawing blood out may indeed cause alarm because once it has been taken out, they believe that there is no way to replace it; hence, an imbalance for life. Multiple blood tests can create anxiety for the Hmong patient and family. In Seng Pao's case, passage of blood from the nasogastric tube was a strong indicator of imminent death to him and his family. Cutting off protective strings (the sicker the person, the more strings), along with the absence of family, may contribute to declining health.

In our story, Seng Pao continues to ask for his wife. Reliance on the comfort and protection of the family during uncertain times of ill health is an expectation, especially during hospitalization. Why is family so important? It is thought that evil spirits and menacing ghosts roam the hallways of the hospital and could bring harm, or even death, to the individual. Family members must remain at the bedside to protect the person from those spirits. Honoring the ill patient helps to ensure that, after death, his or her spirit will protect the family as well as bring good fortune.

The belief in the spirit world is very strong. It is believed that the body has three souls: one that stays with the body; one that goes off to heaven; and one that is reincarnated as a person, animal, or thing. If the first soul wanders, leaving the body at night and failing to return in the morning, the person will become ill (Livo, Cha 1991). Protection is sought against soul loss, which causes illness and stress. Lengthy ceremonies, which may take several days, are used to restore health. These are an integral part of the the Hmong culture. Dabs, malevolent spirits that roam the earth, can snatch a soul, and only with the help of the shaman, also known as txiv neeb, can health be restored. Protective items such as strings worn around the wrist, ankle, or neck can offer protection and keep the soul within the body.

Illness can be of a supernatural nature, and this is thought to be more devastating than illness caused by an imbalance in the Yin and Yang. Soul loss, angry ancestors, and malevolent spirits are considered among the causes of serious illnesses. In each case, the individual is considered to be the victim of an assault from an outside power. Loss occurs when the soul wanders off or becomes separated because of anger, grief, or curiosity or if it is frightened by a sudden noise, as is the case of Lia Lao in Anne Fadiman's book (1996 p. 13). It is believed Lia's soul was snatched by a *dab*. A *neeb*, healing spirit, is then summoned by the *txiv neeb* in shamanic rituals to heal. Animals such as a pig, chicken, or dog are sacrificed during this ceremony to barter for the soul of the sick person. The animal chosen to be sacrificed is based on the animal's ability and strength to fight in the spirit world. Dogs are used for those who are extremely ill, as they are considered the most ferocious and fight the hardest in the spirit world. Contrary to some beliefs, dogs are used rarely and they are not eaten. Sharon Johnson in her article, *Hmong Health Beliefs and Experiences in the Western Health Care System*, describes the ceremonies in which the shaman calls the patient's soul back home:

> Usually, two Shaman ceremonies will be conducted: one when the diagnosis is made, the second when healing occurs. During the first ceremony, the Shaman goes to the spirit world to find out where the soul is and what payment (sacrifice) the soul requires to return to the individual or what must be done to placate the spirit that is causing the illness. During the second ceremony the blood of the animal will be placed on clothing that the ill person wears or on the person's skin.
>
> Johnson (2002 p.128)

The strong belief in the healing powers of the txiv neeb provides assurance that everything is being done to restore the health of the ill person. The position of t*xiv neeb*, similar to other healers such as curandero or hilot, is not a role one chooses, but rather a calling The individual is someone from the community who is well respected and knowledgeable about the spirit world and who treats both the body and the soul. As HCPs, we can extend an invitation to the txiv neeb to collaborate in the healing of a Hmong patient.

Patient education is integral to the healing process as well. Our medical terms do not translate easily, word for word, into the Hmong language. In addition, Hmong people have little knowledge of the anatomy of the body, which creates a barrier to care. Given those two aspects and limited English proficiency, the HCP needs to create patient educational material that is reflective of Hmong beliefs and communication needs. Similar to the diabetic material found in Chapter 14, which uses the symbol of the Medicine Wheel to show the correlation between the value of history (ancestors) and present day diet, educational material in a similar format can be used for the Hmong population. Using symbols found in the Hmong culture facilitates an educational process that is meaningful and easily understandable. Given their oral tradition, story telling and group sharing may be an effective way to lead a discussion about preventative care methods. Learning by doing – actual hands-on activities – is another effective method that is used.

> <u>Reflective exercise</u>: **Understanding the differences**
> 1. *Do spirits make you sick? Cause you harm? Keep you well?*
> 2. *What stories have you heard about the Hmong ceremonies involving animals?*
> 3. *Have you been invited by the family to join in the ceremony?*
> 4. *How would you explain hypertension or diabetes to a Hmong patient?*
> 5. *Have healers been invited to collaborate in the development of educational materials?*
> 6. *What educational material that you currently use would be effective for the Hmong patient? What would you change?*

*   *   *   *

Finding understanding and balance with other cultural groups, such as the Hmong people, may seem like a never-ending challenge, yet each small step we take leads to acceptance of differences, celebration of the similarities, and discovery of common ground. We actually have more in common than one would think, and it is on that premise that we embrace each encounter with respect and dignity.

<h1 align="center">Culture Care Modes & Actions
Hmong – Gastric Bleeding</h1>

Preservation/Maintenance
- Respect for clan leader
- Extended family
- Tradition and history

Accommodation/Negotiation
- Oral tradition
- Folk practices
- Respect for Tvix Neeb

Repatterning/Restructuring
- Explanation of anatomy

*   *   *   *

Engaging in literature . . . An Activity

Anne Fadiman's book, *The Spirit Catches You and You Fall Down*, brings to light the importance of cultural awareness, sensitivity, and competence. It is the story about a Hmong family who fled the mountains of Laos, lived in a refugee camp in Thailand for several years, and then emigrated to the United States, specifically the central valley of California. It revolves around Lia, the three-month-old daughter of the Kao family, who becomes ill and is taken to the emergency room. What ensues is the ongoing misunderstandings between the Kao family and the medical community, leading to tension and frustration.

Literature such as this affords you an opportunity to read about an event that could have happened at your facility, but did not. It is a human portrayal that draws our attention and keeps the reader riveted to the story. Given our medical background, this book challenges us to think of how we might have done things differently. While the story centers on the Hmong culture, it could be any cultural group that is different from our own. It is what we don't know about a person's beliefs, values, and healthcare practices that gets in the way of providing culturally competent care.

In the article, *A Literary Approach to Teaching Cultural Competency* by Clark et al. (2000), the author suggests that we, as healthcare providers (specifically nurses), use the book not only to discuss the Kao family, but also topics such as acculturation, refugees, immigrants, healing ceremonies, and healers. How prepared are we to meet the needs of a diverse society? This book is so highly recommended because it moves us to learn more and to embrace diversity in our everyday experiences. The following questions serve as a discussion guide.

1. Since the events considered in this book unfolded in the 1980's, what has changed?
2. How are nurses, physicians, and other members of the healthcare team portrayed in the book, and what contributions (or mistakes) are attributed to them during the course of their care for Lia Lee and her family?
3. As nurses, we believe we have emerged in the last two centuries from low status, voluntary, and largely invisible laborers to professionals with a disciplinary knowledge base and professional identity. Does Fadiman reflect this same understanding of nursing? What influences in her life as a journalist and nursing outsider might account for her portrayal of the various health professions?

4. What responsibility did the nurses taking care of Lia and the Lee family have for providing, documenting, and communicating their nursing interventions and outcomes? In what ways (if any) are these responsibilities different when we care for patients from culturally diverse backgrounds?

5. In the book, several avenues of action are intimated as being worthwhile in our future healthcare system and programs of professional education to increase accessibility and quality of care across cultural differences. What are these courses of action? What else do you think needs to be improved?

6. How might an effective empowered nurse have changed the course of events in the book? Ideally, what attitudes, knowledge, and skills would this person possess?

7. What aspects of health policy and healthcare delivery need to change to alter the course of care for immigrants and refugees such as the Lee family?

Clark, L., Zuk, J., Baramee, J. (2000 p. 201)
Used with permission

Resources

Andrews, M. M., Boyle, J. S. (2008). *Transcultural concepts in nursing care*. (5th Ed.).New York: Lippincott Williams & Wilkins.

Clark, L., Zuk, J., Baramee, J. (2000). A literary approach to teaching cultural competency. *Journal of Transcultural Nursing*. (11)3, 199-203.

Duffy, J., Harmon, R., Ranard, D. A., Thao, B., Yang, K. (2004). The Hmong: An Introduction to Their History and Culture. Washington DC: Center for Applied Linguistics.

Fadiman, A. (1996). The Spirit Catches You and You Fall Down. New York: Farrar, Straus and Giroux.

Giger, J. N., Davidhizar, R. E. (2008). Transcultural nursing: Assessment and intervention. (5th Ed.).St Louis, MO: Mosby/Elsevier.

Helsel, D., Mochel, M., Bauer, R. (2005). Chronic illness and Hmong shamans. *Journal of Transcultural Nursing*. (16)2, 150-154.

Helsel, D., Mochel, M. (2002). Afterbirths in the afterlife: Culture meaning of placenta disposal in a Hmong-American community. *Journal of Transcultural Nursing*. (13)4, 282-286.

Hodge, F. S., Pasqua, B. A., Marquez, C. A., Cantrell, B. G. (2001). Utilizing traditional storytelling to promote wellness in American Indian communities. *Journal of Transcultural Nursing*. 13(1), 6-11.

Johnson, S. K. (2002). Hmong health beliefs and experiences in western health care system. *Journal of Transcultural Nursing*. (13)2, 126-132.

Leininger, M. M. (1991). Culture care diversity and universality: A theory of nursing. New York: National League for Nursing Press.

Leininger, M. M., McFarland, M. R. (2002). Transcultural nursing: Concepts, theories, research and practice. (3rd Ed.). New York: McGraw-Hill.

Lipson, J. G., Dibble, S. L., (2005). Culture & Clinical Care. San Francisco CA: UCSF Nursing Press.

McGoldrick, M, Giordano, J., Garcia-Preto, N. (2005). *Ethnicity & Family Therapy*. (3rd Ed.). New York: Guilford Press

McClain-Ruelle, L., Xiong, K. (2005). Continuing the promise: Recruiting and preparing Hmong-American educators for Central Wisconsin. *Hmong Studies Journal*. Volume 6, p.1-16.

Ramsey, J. G. (2001). A contradiction of cultural conservatism. *Education Week*. (21)4, 37.

Vue, X. (2005). Working with Hmong: A communication and orality paradigm. Retrieved on October 1, 2009, from www.dhs.state.mn.us

Warner, M. E., Mochel, M. (1998). The Hmong and health care in Merced, California. *Hmong Studies Journal*. (2)2, 1-30.

The Power Of Prayer . . .

Let The Healing Begin!

(African American)

16

I know I'm okay now . . .

Mother Powell tries to stretch. Her left side seems to move just fine, but the voices of her congregation are coming from the other direction. She can hear Sister Elmyra – she couldn't miss that deep raspy throat, and Pastor Grant, with his even more thunderous tones – their voices raised so that it's almost like preaching. But the nurses don't seem to be listening.

"Woe to the ones who keep the shepherd from his flock, the woman from her sister! – The voice of God will speak, calling upon you to have faith, to let her church family into the room to lay hands on her. God will make things right as rain, as the lilies in the field – the meek will inherit . . ."

Mother Powell isn't sure that she is hearing the words, but she feels buoyed, held aloft by the very presence of her people.

"So why can't they come in?" she thinks.

She keeps trying to move her right side so that she can see over in the direction where the sounds are coming.

"Leaning, leaning, safe and secure from all alarms, leaning, leaning, leaning on the the Everlasting Arms."

Mother Powell is a big woman, thin-legged but carrying a bit too much "junk in the trunk," as she's heard it called. Quite a bit up front too. She doesn't know what happened to her this morning, just that she was fixing the flowers in the sanctuary when all of a sudden everything went blank. The next thing she knew here she was in the hospital.

"I won't have this predicament set me back. The prayer warriors at Calvary Baptist need me."

Mother Powell finds that she can hum. She starts with a single note only,

191

loud and insistent. When that doesn't seem to bring any attention from the nurses, she hums even more loudly, one hymn after another.
  "God's eye is on the sparrow and I know He watches me."

*   *   *   *

History . . . Family . . . Religion

It's not just religion; it's spirituality and a belief in something greater that oneself – something to rely upon in times of crisis, illness, and death. Church members bring comfort, assurance, care, and presence. Help is simply a phone call away. The African-American church provides a foundation of support. It is a sanctuary, a place of worship, and most importantly, a community.

With the end of the Civil War and the passage of the 13th, 14th, and 15th amendments, slavery was abolished. The right to vote, own property, and serve on a jury were established. With the freedom to assemble without fear of retribution, change came. African-American churches and schools were established. Leaders emerged. Three hundred years of slavery preceded this time. Extended family, highly valued in the African-American community, and spirituality were the foundation that enabled them to face each day and live through the atrocities of slavery. Lascelles Black (2004) writes, "Living with the constant threat of separation and loss through the sale of a family member by a white master, the family sustained itself by placing a high value on each member, no matter how distant the blood relationship may be" (p. 59).

What could not be taken away were beliefs and values about family and spirituality. Each serves as a foundation that has enabled African-Americans to face each day and live through the atrocities of slavery. Lascelles Black (2004) writes, "Living with the constant threat of separation and loss through the sale of a family member by a white master, the family sustained itself by placing a high value on each member, no matter how distant the blood relationship may be" (p. 59). This extended family, highly valued in the African culture, would continue to be an integral part of the African-American life.

At an exhibit at the de Young Museum in San Francisco in the spring of 2007, a group of African-American women from Gee's Bend, Alabama, talked about families being separated during slavery. The *Quiltmakers of Gee's Bend*, as they have come to be known, told their story that began on a plantation in North Carolina in the mid 1800s. Falling on hard times, the master sold one hundred slaves. Alonzio Pettway shared that her grandmother, who arrived in 1859, was "bought and for a dime." She remembers her grandmother saying, "I never saw my mother or brother again." Forced to migrate (on foot) over 1,000 miles to Gee's Bend, Alabama, life continued to be a struggle. One aspect that sustained them during this time was religion. The church was a place of support, community, and hope. It provided when nothing else did.

Prejudice and discrimination followed the end of the Civil War and perpetuated the cycle of poverty. Separation was the policy. Economic opportunities were limited, especially in the South. The 1940s saw a large migration of Blacks to the North in search of a better life without fear of violence. My friend, James, an elderly African-American gentleman who was part of our church community, told about a lynching that took place in the 1930s when he was seventeen and living in the south. He showed us a newspaper clipping of two young men hanging by the neck with a third noose dangling free. "That one was suppose to be me, but I got away." He continued to be haunted by that experience.

Out of the church came leadership. One leader, in particular, was the Reverend Martin Luther King Jr. Using the established churches and their leadership as the base, he brought awareness of the injustices experienced by the African-American population, regardless of its geographic location. In turn, his message inspired others to join the movement that eventually brought about the Civil Rights Act of 1964 and the Voting Rights Act of 1965. Separate but equal was no longer the mantra. Yet, the struggle continues.

Healthcare Disparities . . .

Mistrust of the healthcare system plays a role in access to care and treatment for persons of color. When the statistics are tallied, it is apparent that African-Americans are at a higher risk of developing and dying from heart disease, stroke, breast cancer, and childbirth. The documentary, *Unnatural Causes: Is Inequality Making Us Sick?* (2008), posits that an increase in stress due to discrimination has an effect on the body. Relentless exposure to racism over months and years can cause the body to produce high levels of cortisol which, in turn, increases blood pressure and glucose. The result is a lowering of the immune system and an acceleration of the aging process.

Economics and education also affect health outcomes. Twenty-two percent of African-Americans live at or below the poverty level. The Civil Rights Report of 2004 indicates an annual dropout rate of fifty percent for African-American high school students. Together, these statistics contribute to poor health. Is the problem access to care, socioeconomic issues, educational discrepancies, or lack of trust for the healthcare system? It may be a combination of all four of these. However, we need to consider history: Starting in the late 1800s, there was segregation by the American Medical Association with the establishment of "colored" hospitals. This sent a clear message. It would take another century to eliminate this overt discrimination against African-Americans.

Cultural beliefs and values

Values and beliefs, such as family ties and religion, sustain people during difficult times. We can see from our story that Mother Powell, ailing in her hospital bed, hears her "sisters in Christ" and her pastor just outside the door. She finds this a source of strength and reassurance. She hums her favorite songs and quotes scripture. She relies on what is familiar to her and this gives her a sense of peace and hope. Ethnostudies done by Dr. Leininger and others identified cultural care values found in the African-American population including the following:

African-American Cultural Beliefs & Values
- Extended family networks
- Religion valued
- Interdependence
- Folk food
- Folk healing modes
- Music and physical activity

Dr Leininger (1991 p. 357)

Extended family may include people who are not blood related but are considered part of the family and are treated as such. They provide support: physically, emotionally, and spiritually. Sunday dinners, reunions, and celebrations provide venues for gathering together and establish a sense of identity and belonging. One can always count on the extended family to be there when needed. Interdependence is not considered reciprocal, but rather open and fluid. Meeting needs as they arise without being concerned about future payments is the value.

For many African-Americans, the church community is a place of religion, spirituality, and fellowship. "Prayer warriors," as I knew them when living in Wisconsin, were indeed a powerful group of women who could be counted on in times of illness, life-threatening conditions, and crises to intercede on behalf of the individual or family. For the recipient of the prayers, this brought assurance that the current difficulties could indeed be overcome. On many occasions these "warriors," came to the hospital where I worked to lay hands on, pray, and sing with the patient. As HCPs, we need to accommodate and welcome people from the church. In doing so, we may even have the opportunity to witness healing.

Music is interwoven into the African-American culture. During slavery, music and song were a part of the church services, used in community gatherings and used to signal that an impending escape was to take place. Spirituals, such as "Steal Away", "Wade in the Water" or the "Chariots a Comin" would be used to send particular messages. Today, music continues to be an integral part of African-

American life. In Ken Burn's series, *History of Jazz*, he highlights the influence of African and European music to create the "art of jazz."

Like music, folk healing practices have been passed down from generation to generation within the African-American community. In addition to religious rituals, treatments include both folk practices and western medicine. Granny healers may be deemed shamans. They are called on to care for individuals and employ remedies such as herbal teas and poultices.

<u>Reflective exercise</u>: **The value of culture**
1. *How are your cultural values and beliefs different from the African-American culture?*
2. *Where do you find common ground?*
3. *How could these beliefs and values be incorporated into appointments, treatment plans, and conversation?*

Communication . . . it's a part of me

...and how I reveal myself to others. As one African-American social worker from New York shared at one of my seminars, "I speak Black English at home and Standard English in the workplace." Black English, also know as Ebonics, is a dialect of the English language. Pronunciation of words, as well as grammar and sentence structure, are different. For example, dropping the final "*g*" in the word "talking," it now becomes "*talkin*," and going becomes "*goin*." A concluding "*f*" could take the place of "th" as in the word "*wif*" instead of "*with*." The use of this dialect does not necessarily equate to socioeconomic or educational status. It is important that the HCP acknowledge this fact and avoid possible stereotyping based on the use of language. Black English, as the seminar participant suggested, is used socially in the African-American community and should not be considered substandard or incorrect. Rather, it provides a structure that supports cultural and ethnic identity (Cherry, Giger 2008, p. 194).

Expressive and dynamic in elocution, the African-American patient may seem overly emotional or intrusive to a HCP who is not familiar with this style of communication. The tone of voice conveys the message. Facial and hand gestures emphasize the point of the communiqué. In her book, *Culturally Responsive Teaching*, Geneva Gay (2000) cites researchers in the field of education who posit "African-Americans (especially those most strongly affiliated with their ethnic identity and cultural heritage) tend to take positions of advocacy and express personal points of view in discussions . . . the worth of a particular line of reasoning is established by challenging the validity of oppositional ideas and by the level of personal ownership of the individuals" (p.100). Silence, on the other hand, may send a message of disagreement or distrust.

195

Eye contact is vital, demonstrating respect and engagement in the conversation. An African-American nurse at a community hospital shared, "If I didn't look my grandmother in the eye, she thought I was lying." Another item to note is that in some cases a word conveys a different meaning. For example, if something is bad it may really mean good. Taking medication behind a meal may mean it is taken after a meal. One of my patients talked about carrying his daughter to the appointment. That meant that he drove her to the clinic.

When responding to questions by the HCP, the patient may use a narrative approach: the story, the circumstances surrounding the event, the people involved, the treatments tried, and the results. The HCP, on the other hand, may use a linear approach, wanting to know just the facts: onset of symptoms and current health status, for example. Allowing time to listen leads to a better understanding of the patient's perception of the illness. In reality, listening takes less time and establishes more trust than rushing someone through an appointment.

Time . . . is not of the essence

Time is generally more circular than linear in the African-American culture; flexibility and attention to the moment rather than arriving at the designated time afford a more relaxed approach. Present day orientation, thought to be the more dominant time frame, does not negate the importance and effect of past events or future aspirations. One way in which many African-Americans are future oriented is when considering their own deaths. For at least one African-American elderly woman, it was crucial to make all payments toward her funeral expenses. Her granddaughter shared that there were times when she did not pay the electric bill in order to ensure enough money to pay her life insurance.

Planning for the future, on the other hand, may seem futile for some African-Americans when considering the effects of prejudice, discrimination, and racism on their socioeconomic and educational opportunities. One only need contemplate the low rate of high school graduation, coupled with high unemployment and poverty levels, to validate this concept. Education, however, is valued highly in the African-American family; it ensures future well-being. Children are encouraged to do well in school, as that sets the stage for future socioeconomic stability.

Family . . . is everything

Historically in Africa, families were close, connected, and organized to serve the needs of all. Everything changed in 1619 with the beginning of what would be more than three hundred years of slavery. The subjugation of the slaves by plantation owners had a devastating effect on family life. Marriages were banned and children were the property of the slave owner. Husbands were unable to provide protection or security for their families. Even after emancipation, African-American men were denied employment or relegated to dehumanizing jobs, further weakening the stability of the family. Extended families, therefore, became the source of security and reliability, and continue to be an integral part of the African-American culture.

The African-American family of the 21st century can be patriarchal or matriarchal. According the the U.S. Department of Health and Human Services (2006), forty-four percent of all black household are headed by women. In a matriarchal family, the aunts, grandmothers, and other women provide financial, emotional, and physical support. If the family is patriarchal, responsibilities and roles are more egalitarian. Women are generally the ones who ensure the health of all family members by attending appointments and advocating for the individual. However, this does not mean that they are the sole decision maker. It is important for the HCP to include the African-American man as well. Inquiring how decisions are made in the family with regard to health is one way to understand family structure.

Older African-American women are held in high esteem and are respected for their insight and wisdom, especially during illness. They provide stability to the home, and at times are the caregivers when parents work. It is important for the HCP to ask how they would like to be addressed and to listen to their opinions.

African-American children are expected to show respect for their parents and elders, do well in school, and help out at home. Respectful behavior is requested. The firm discipline of the parent provides a stable and loving environment, and support from the family ensures the child's future.

Reflective exercise: the family
1. *How has your history influenced your family structure? The role of women? The role of men?*
2. *Do you inquire of your patient how decisions are made within the family?*
3. *Who is part of that decision-making process?*
4. *Do you address the elderly as Mr., Mrs., or Ms? or by their first name?*

Health beliefs – church as educational opportunity

Health for African-Americans may be described as feeling well and living in harmony with their surroundings. Illness may be due to natural causes such as improper diet, stress, or exposure to elements of cold or heat. Supernatural causes include conflict or disharmony with relationships as punishment from God for bad behavior or the affliction of bad spirits. One colleague shared with us that "she was exhausted and unable to get out of bed." The cause: God wanted her to listen to His message and she never stopped to listen. Perception of the cause of an illness is one's personal reality. Our responsibility is to ask the question: What do you think caused your illness?

The African-American patient may not seek professional care initially, but instead use home remedies first. In the movie *Soul Food*, the matriarch inadvertently burns her arm. Her daughters race to assist her informing her that she needs to see a doctor because she has diabetes and the burn could lead to a serious infection. She resists that notion and states: "I don't need to see a doctor. There is nothing that a little of my herbs and salve won't cure." Because she is still able to continue her daily activities, she sees no need to seek care. An inability to fulfill one's obligations to work may be the first acknowledgment of illness.

Health beliefs and practices of the African-American community may include all of the aforementioned approaches: biomedicine, naturalistic, and personalistic, as discussed in Chapter 9. Treatments can include medication prescribed by their healthcare provider as well as teas, herbs, and poultices suggested by folk healers. I lived in the same neighborhood as Ms. Anne. She was a quiet, unassuming woman who imparted health advice to those who lived around her. If ever there were problems, neighbors would always say, "Go see Miss Anne." It was tacitly understood: she was the healer.

In some rural areas, magic or voodoo may be practiced in the African-American population. Within the church community, laying on of hands and prayer circles are common. As we can see from our vignette, the church ladies and the pastor are at the hospital, ready to provide healing through faith and prayer. For Mother Powell, her faith and the presence of the believers assure that she is not alone and that whatever comes, she will be able to face it.

> **Reflective exercise: Faith and Healing**
> 1. *How are faith communities welcomed into the healthcare setting?*
> 2. *Does your belief system include faith healing, laying on of hands, or prayer circles?*
> 3. *Are herbs and folks healers part of your belief and culture?*
> 4. *In what ways are you the same as or different from Mother Powell?*
> 5. *How do you welcome faith communities into the healthcare setting?*

Religion & Community

Eric Lincoln (1984), a theologian and historian of the African-American church in America, stated: "To understand the power of the African-American church, it must first be understood that there is no distinction between the African-American church and the Black community. The Church is the spiritual face of Black subculture, and whether one is a member or not is beside the point" (p.96).

Pastor C provides an afterschool homework program for the members of his congregation and anyone else who would like to participate. He attended several parent-teacher conferences at the local elementary school. The principal finally asked who he was. He replied, "I am the pastor of the church and these students attend our afterschool program. If they aren't doing well, I want to know." He became the link between the school and the community, making sure that "his" children received the education they needed.

As HCPs we can set up an outreach connection with the church community. Establishing rapport with the Pastor and church members opens a dialogue that can lead to a more trusting relationship. Endorsement by members who had a positive experience with a HCP encourages others to seek care. In addition, the church can sponsor a health fair or invite guest speakers to address the health concerns of a member. A colleague told about a group of African-American women with breast cancer who shared their story during the service at the local churches. Using the oral tradition of storytelling, these women were able to reach others within their community and encourage them to seek preventative care including pap smears and mammograms.

Reflective exercise: Religion and Health Practices
1. *Do outreach programs in your organization include the churches in your area?*
2. *Are community ministers and pastors part of the pastoral team?*
3. *Are pastors and church leaders consulted in the development of policies?*

*   *   *   *

Mother Powell knows that, for her, belief in God and membership in her church will sustain her during hospitalization. The presence of the extended family in the Intensive Care Unit waiting room along with immediate family may be overwhelming to the hospital staff, but the HCP can ask: "Who is the spokesperson?" Then working with that person, develop a plan that assures that all who come are welcome to visit with the patient. Creating a welcoming environment sends the message that you care, understand, and respect the importance of extended family.

Culture Care Modes & Actions
African-American – Hospitalization

Preservation/Maintenance
- Respect for elderly
- Religious beliefs and practices

Accommodation/Negotiation
- Visitation of extended family
- Religious rituals – healing and prayer
- Folk practices – herbal teas

Repatterning/Restructuring
- Diet and exercise

Resources

Andrews. M. M. (2008). Religion, culture and nursing. In Andrews, M. M., Boyle, J. S. (Eds.) *Transcultural Concepts in Nursing.* Care. (5th Ed.). Philadelphia: Lippincott.

Campinha-Bacote, J. (2008). People of African American heritage. In Purnell, L. D., Paulanka, B. J. (Eds.) Transcultural Health Care: A Culturally Competent Approach. (3rd Ed.). Philadelphia PA: F. A. Davis.

Carey, C., Osborne, H., Veatch, D. (2004). The Quiltmakers of Gee's Bend. Alabama: Alabama State Council on the Arts.

Cherry, B., Giger, J. N. (2008). African Americans. In Giger, J. N., Davidhizar, R. E. (Eds.) Transcultural Nursing: Assessment and Intervention. (5th Ed.) St Louis, MO: Mosby/Elsevier.

Gay, G. (2000). Culturally Responsive Teaching: Theory, Research & Practice. New York: Teachers College Press.

Giger, J. N., Appel, S. J., Davidhizar, R. E., Davis, C. (2008). Church and spirituality in the lives of the African American community. *Journal of Transcultural Nursing.* (19)4, 375-383.

Graham-Garcia, J., Raines, T. L., Andrews, J. O., Mensah, G. A. (2001). Race, ethnicity, and geography disparities in heart disease in women of color. *Journal of Transcultural Nursing.* (12)1, 56-67.

Hines, P. M., Boyd-Franklin, N.. (2005). African American Families. In McGoldrick, M., Giordano, J. Garcia-Preto, N. (Eds) *Ethnicity & Family Therapy.* (3rd Ed.). New York: Guilford Press

Leininger, M. M. (1991). Culture care diversity and universality: A theory of nursing. New York: National League for Nursing Press.

Leininger, M. M., McFarland, M. R. (2002). Transcultural nursing: Concepts, theories, research and practice. (3rd Ed.). New York: McGraw-Hill.

Lincoln, E. (1984). Race, religion, and the Continuing American Dilemma. New York: Hill and Wang.

Locks. S., Waters, C.M. (2005). African Americans. In Lipson, J. G., Dibble, S. L., (Eds.) Culture & Clinical Care. San Francisco CA: UCSF Nursing Press.

Loeb, S. J., (2006). African American older adults coping with chronic health conditions. *Journal of Transcultural Nursing.* (17)2, 139-147.

Nelms, L. W., Gorski, J. (2006). The role of the African traditional healer in women's health. *Journal of Transcultural Nursing.* (17)2, 184-189.

Penner, L. A., Dovidio, J. F., Edmondson, D., Dailey, R. K., Markova, T., Albrecht, T. L., Gaertner, S. L. (2009). The experience of discrimination and Black-White health disparities in medical care. *Journal of Black Psychology.* (35)2, 181-203.

Plowden, K. O., Wenger, A. F. Z. (2001). Stranger to friend enabler: Creating a community of caring in African American research using ethnonursing methods. *Journal of Transcultural Nursing.* (12)1, 34-39.

Ramer, L., Richardson, J. L., Cohen, M. Z., Bedney, C., Danley, K. L., Judge, E. A. (1999). Multimeasure pain assessment in an ethnically diverse group of patients with cancer. *Journal of Transcultural Nursing.* (10)2, 94-101.

Savage, C. L., Anthony, J., Lee, R., Kappesser, M. L., Rose, B. (2007). The culture of pregnancy and infant care in African American women: An ethnographic study. *Journal of Transcultual Nursing.* (18)3, 215-223.

Shusta, R. M., Levine, D. R., Wong, H. Z., Olson, A. T., Harris, P. R. (2008). *Multicultural Law Enforcement: Strategies for Peacekeeping in a Diverse Society.* (4th Ed.) New Jersey: Pearson, Prentice Hall.

Spector, R. (2009). *Cultural diversity in health and illness.* (7th Ed.), New Jersey: Pearson/Prentice Hall.

U.S. Department of Health and Human Services, Health Resources and Services Administration, Women's Health USA 2006. Rockville, Maryland: U.S. Department of Health and Human Services, 2006.

Wisneski, L. A., Anderson, L. (2005). The Scientific Basis of Integrative Medicine.New York: CRC Press.

Can You Feel My Pain . . .

(Vietnamese)

17

"Make them stop poking me, Mommy. Make them take out this thing in my arm. It Huuuuuurts!"

Matthew, age seven, has just had surgery on a broken leg. He is wiggling all over the bed as his mother, Kathleen, wrings her hands by his side. Occasionally she leans down to make sure he doesn't pull out the tube which, she assumes, must be the antibiotics or at least something to make her little boy better. She herself can not accomplish that. The doctors were very skilled, she's sure, and Matthew does have a lovely room as hospitals go, light and not too noisy. Matthew on the other hand, is loud.

"Owwwww! Why don't you help me, Mommy? My leg hurts and my arm hurts and I have to pee. Owwwww."

Lau Xuan comes into the room, having heard the commotion from the other end of the hallway. She frowns slightly, using all her will not to. She readjusts the tube, looking away from Mrs. Riley due to respect, and from Matthew due to an overwhelming feeling of dislike. She can't help herself.

"Who does he think he is anyway? He has just had excellent medical care from top surgeons. He has hs own bed. He seems healthy otherwise. Why is he yelling at all the people who are trying to help him?"

Lau Xuan thinks of her own family, her well-behaved sisters and brothers. Well, sometimes the boys caused a little trouble, probably following in the footsteps of their schoolmates in this country. But certainly they wouldn't have gotten away with any disrespect in Vietnam. Harmony was paramount.

Lau Xuan had been pretty brave to decide on nursing school. She's the first in her family to have gone to college and she knows that her parents and her grandmother are proud of her. Her grandparents had fled to this country in 1972 in the midst of the American War, but her grandfather died shortly afterwards.

She was his special favorite and she knows that he would have been especially delighted; Lau Xuan had worked hard and succeeded.

"So who is this boy Matthew? Why does he think he can complain when so many other people have been hurt so much more?"

Lau Xuan remembers her instructor, Mrs. Southern, cautioning her the other day when she was upset by a little girl brought into emergency, one who had been protesting ever since they wheeled her through the doors. But all Mrs. Southern had said was to "Deal with it." What Lau Xuan had wanted to do was to tell the girl to be quiet, not to yell at the nurses and especially not at her father. She remembered looking in amazement at the man and the concern in his eyes for his daughter. He had just stood there taking the abuse from his child.

"What a little brat," she thought. "Certainly have seen some examples of American brats since I've been working in pediatrics. What am I not getting?"

*   *   *   *

The issues in this vignette highlight two of Lau's cultural belief and values: respect for authority and response to pain. She finds herself caught between her expectations and the reality of the clinical situation. She expects the mother to intervene and quiet the child, and she expects her nursing instructor to support her in this process. Respect for those in authority and avoidance of conflict are among Lau's cultural beliefs, yet in this situation she realizes that these may not be shared by her clinical instructor or by the parent. Ethnically diverse students may have had similar experiences, which may lead to misunderstanding and conflict.

Three waves . . . the formation of community in the United States

It's 1952. The setting is Saigon, Vietnam. An English newsman (Michael Caine) encounters Arie Powell (Jeb Bentin) at a local cafe. It is not coincidence that brings them together. *The Quiet American*, later made into a movie, was written in 1958 by Graham Greene. It centers on the story of the Vietnamese national liberation movement for control of the then existing French colony. It sets the stage for what was to come: the Vietnam War or, according to my Vietnamese friend, the American War. It depends on one's perspective.

Vietnam's history fluctuates between independence and colonization. Following domination by the Chinese for over a thousand years, Vietnam enjoyed nine hundred years of independence before colonization by France in 1858. What followed was the Indochina War, which ended French occupation. The Geneva Accord of 1954 split Vietnam along the 17th parallel, North and South Vietnam, with Russian support in the North and American in the South.

What began as assistance by the Americans in the form of military advisors in the early 1960s escalated into a full conflict which ended in 1975. Following thirty years of war, Vietnam was devastated physically, socially, and environmentally. Thus began migration to other countries. The first wave of emigrants to the United States began in 1975. These individuals were generally professionals, high ranking military, and families from wealthy backgrounds who often spoke English. Their ability to acculturate to their host country, the United States, was directly related to their ability to secure employment. The second wave of immigrants began in 1978 and these people came to be known as *"the boat people."* Seeking freedom, they left under duress and pressure from the newly formed South Vietnamese government. Less educated and in poor physical condition, the boat people found acculturation slow in coming. What support there was came in the form of close-knit Vietnamese communities already established in America. The third wave titled the *"Orderly Departure Program"* began in 1979 and provided safe and legal exit for persons wanting to unite with their families in America. A fourth wave, occasioned by the "Amerasian Homecoming Act" in 1987, offered entry for military officers, political detainees, children of American serviceman, Vietnamese women, and their close relatives.

With each succeeding generation, the Vietnamese people have contributed to the rich diversity found in the United States. Through cultural values of hard work, family loyalty, and education such as Lua's nursing program, they established a willingness to participate and engage in this new life.

Cultural beliefs . . . make dreams a reality

Lua Xuan's belief in hard work and respect for elders and those in authority provides the foundation for her to excel in the academic and clinical settings. We can see, however, from her story that these beliefs may be in conflict with those of her instructor and possibly the child's parent. The following cultural care beliefs and values cited by Dr. Madeleine Leininger and others are from Vietnamese refugees living in the United States.

Vietnamese Cultural Values & Beliefs
- Harmony and balance in universe
- Extended kinship family ties
- Religious and spiritual values
- Respect for elderly and authority
- Folk care practice
- Food and environment

Leininger (et al. 2004 p 360)

Vietnamese culture was heavily influenced by China due to nine hundred years of occupation. The adoption of Confucianism from the Chinese brought with it values of harmony and balance along with respect for the universe, parents, and those who teach. Minimizing self and acknowledging the importance of the group highlights the value of avoiding conflict and confrontation, thus maintaining self-esteem and harmony in all relationships. Forgiveness is readily available in order to resolve issues that lead to tension. Family loyalty is the foundation.

> **Reflective exercise: Values we hold . . .**
> 1. *What has been your experience with Vietnamese colleagues, patients, and community?*
> 2. *How are your values different from theirs?*
> 3. *Where do you find common ground?*
> 4. *Where do you think tensions might arise in the workforce?*

Family

"Filial piety" commands respect and obedience from children to their parents. The Vietnamese family is hierarchal and patriarchal, with the father as head of the household. Decision-making is usually done by the father or the eldest son. Gender roles are well defined, with the husband as provider and the wife as the caregiver and nurturer. Again this is changing for some families who have resided in the United States for a longer period of time and whose socioeconomic and educational levels are higher. Role reversal actually began years before emigration when war and economic conditions forced the wife to seek outside employment in Vietnam.

Children, highly valued in Vietnamese society, are protected and sheltered. They are taught to be respectful and obedient to the parents and elders. As Lua noted earlier, Vietnamese children are also taught to be honest, quiet, and polite; bad behavior is thought to affect the family in negative ways. There is a strong emphasis on learning. Success in education reflects positively on the family and assures that the parents are taken care of in their old age.

Elders are afforded respect by all members of the family and are consulted on important decisions. In addition to providing childcare when both parents work, they provide children with an understanding of the Vietnamese cultural beliefs and values of Vietnam. Adjustment to a new country and the Western influence on the children of individualism and assertiveness may cause stress in the relationship. Yet the values of harmony and family prevail to provide the foundation for Vietnamese community.

Communication — Time and Space

As we know, communication is key to understanding. Since Vietnam was occupied by China, France, and America, the population may speak Chinese, French, and/or English in addition to Vietnamese. The Vietnamese language is monosyllabic and includes vowels that use tonal variation to indicate a specific meaning for a word.

Respect and politeness are shown using specific words and avoidance of eye contact. Outside of the family structure, a patient may be soft spoken, showing minimal facial expression. Self control is highly valued, thus expression of emotions may be seen as a sign of weakness. Negative emotions are conveyed by silence or a reluctant smile. Silence and avoidance of eye contact may also be used to avoid disagreement and to maintain a respectful relationship. The values of maintaining harmony and avoiding conflict may lead a patient to answer "yes" when the answer is "no."

Approaching each encounter in a quiet unhurried manner, and addressing the eldest person first, demonstrates respect. While men may shake hands, women do not, and it is best to await the extension of a hand by the patient before offering yours. Speaking softly and using eye contact sparingly helps establish rapport. Beckoning someone to come using a pointed finger is considered an insult, a slightly bowed head as a nod may be a better option.

Time . . .

Past, present, and future time orientation are part of the Vietnamese culture and are influenced by the concept of cycles found in the Buddhist tradition. There is less attention to detail than to exact dates of birth or age. One patient shared that all her siblings' birthdays are celebrated in January regardless of the actual month they were born. Even after death, ancestors continue to be part of the family, providing guidance and protection. There is a strong motivation to please ancestors and keep their memories alive.

Present orientation, an appreciation for the "here and now," may relate to time spent in refugee camps. Present day, at that time, was all about survival. It was a day-to-day existence with no guarantee of immigration to a host country. Yet sharing stories of the long, brutal days in the refugee camp with little shelter, food, or medical care serve as a motivator of hope for the future. Tomorrow was about leaving the camps. Today, future is related to educational and socioeconomic opportunities. In the religious view, future orientation includes education and the anticipation of heaven (Catholic influence) or reincarnation (Buddhist influence).

Health beliefs and practices

Following the second wave of immigration, HCPs in the U.S. were shocked to see ecchymotic areas on the neck and back of children. Thinking that this was child abuse, Child Protective Services became involved. The dilemma for the HCP included a language barrier and a lack of knowledge about the Vietnamese cultural healthcare practices of coining and cupping (described in Chapter 9), both thought to release wind and to restore balance in the body.

Western healthcare may not be sought by the Vietnamese until symptoms become severe. Causes of illness are understood as a natural occurrence, the Chinese influence of Yin and Yang, the wind getting inside the body, and exposure to elements of cold and wind. Supernatural causes include the belief that illness is a result of God's punishment for violation of a societal norm or an angry ancestor.

Prior to the first visit with a HCP, a patient may have seen a traditional healer and used folk practices such as coining, cupping, acupuncture, or other herbal remedies. The role of the sick person, in addition to being stoic in the face of pain, is to maintain a passive role permitting others to care for them. Allowing oneself to regress and be dependent on others is the standard. Family members, including extended family, have the responsibility to provide for the patient's every need. This custom may be in direct contrast to the practices in a Western hospital environment in which self-care is encouraged. Collaboration with the patient and family to incorporate both world views helps to assure a good outcome.

Mental illness may present in the form of somatic complaints. As with many other cultural groups, there is a stigma attached to the admission of a mental or emotional problem. In assessing a patient with mental illness, the HCP needs to consider the individual's history. Even though it may have been twenty or thirty years since immigrating to the United States, memories of war and experiences in the refugee camp may surface unexpectedly. What did this person encounter during the war years? Did they lose family members during the war? Did they spend time in a refugee camp? Do they have flashbacks, nightmares, trouble with insomnia? All of these factors may be indicators of post traumatic stress disorder, depression, anxiety, or all three. When it appears there is no relief to the somatic complaints, it may be time to discuss psychological issues. Hopefully, by this time a trusting relationship has been established enabling the patient and his family to speak freely and openly about this painful experience.

Pain, also known in Vietnamese as dau, is managed in a stoic manner. The pain is no less than that experienced by others, but the outward expression is minimal. Consequently, it may be difficult to ascertain the degree of pain the individual is experiencing. The HCP can use the facial expression chart, which requires the patient to point to which face reflects the degree of pain. Assessment and management of pain from a cultural perspective should be part of the conversation.

Pain . . . a culture response as well

My sister Dee moans when she has pain. I, on the other hand, am very stoic. Our mother is Irish, our father German. I asked her one day why she moans when she is sick. Her response: "Because Mom does and she says she feels better when she moans." I am my father's daughter, quiet and self controlled. Well, not really. I may give the impression that I am strong and can handle pain, and that Dee is weak, but the reality is that we both have pain. We just exhibit it differently.

As a HCP, if you were to encounter us, which one would you think was having more discomfort? Does your response to pain influence how you assess pain in others? Do previous encounters with certain ethnic groups predict your response? Awareness of stereotypes such as "the complaining Jew," the "dramatic and expressive Italians," or the "stoic Asians" should not influence your assessment of the patient's pain. While we would like to think we evaluate each patient as an individual, we must realize that constant exposure to patients' complaints of pain may decrease our sensitivity.

In our story, Lua's assessment of the seven-year-old child's pain is based on the Vietnamese belief that one should be stoic, especially when in a public setting. Matthew, on the other hand, expresses his pain openly and expressively, which is consistent with his family of origin. Lau's expectation that "if the mother would just exercise some control over the child, things would be different" is also consistent with her view of parental responsibility. Pain, thought to be a "physiological phenomenon," actually evokes different expressions and has different meanings for various cultural groups. We learn what is an acceptable response or reaction to pain within our own groups.

Cultural expressions of pain may specify:
- What treatment to seek
- What intensity and duration of pain that should be tolerated
- What responses should be made
- To whom to report when pain occurs
- What types of pain require attention

Meinhart and McCaffery 1983

Every individual, every cultural group, and every religious group may answer those six questions differently. Why and how does the patient respond to pain? Are there overt signs, such as moaning or crying? There are tools that can be used, such as the Likert scale (numbered one to ten with ten being the worst pain) and the facial chart (a continuum of faces from smiling to crying), to determine the depth of pain the patient is experiencing.

209

What are the traditional ways in which comfort is given? It may be in the form of a medication, a cool or hot washcloth on the forehead, a cup of hot tea, or (as in our vignette) direct comfort from mother to child. Many times it is the presence of a family member, a friend, a church member, or a religious leader that brings comfort during a difficult time.

> **Reflective exercise**: **Response to discomfort and pain**
> 1. *How do you express discomfort or pain?*
> 2. *Is it acceptable for you to show pain?*
> 3. *What are some of the comfort measures that help you deal with the pain?*
> 4. *Do you think your cultural views on pain influence your interpretation about others' responses?*
> 5. *Where do you find common ground?*

Health Occupation Faculty . . . those teachable moments

We cannot avoid discussion of minority students in health occupation careers and the importance of culturally competent faculty to address issues of diversity in the healthcare setting. Lau comes to nursing with her cultural beliefs, values, and health practices as she knows them. Perhaps the clinical instructor "does not know that she does not know" about the influence of other cultures on health. This can be a teachable moment. Cultural awareness education for faculty (Chapter 23) ensures a future in which all, students and faculty, have a greater awareness of the importance of culturally sensitive and competent healthcare.

> **Reflective exercise**: **Addressing the situation from student's perspective . . .**
> 1. *Does Lau realize her bias about her patient's response to pain?*
> 2. *What other responses could the clinical instructor offer?*
> 3. *What effect do you think Lau has on the patient and parent?*
> 4. *What strategies could she have used?*

Each patient encounter is unique and offers a learning opportunity, an "aha moment," in which we gain insight into the patient's cultural world. It is essential to ask Lau about her beliefs surrounding response to pain and discuss other clinical experiences that may be related: how were they the same or different. It may be helpful for the instructor to share her experiences as well.

* * * *

Lau Xuan's beliefs and values, passed down from generation to generation, influence her perception of a clinical situation and affect the actions she may take. A culturally knowledgeable and astute faculty member can facilitate a discussion that leads to a broader perspective for Lau Xuan as she cares for patients from diverse ethnic groups. These dialogs, which hopefully include other students, sets the stage for graduating nurses to provide culturally sensitive and competent health care.

Culture Care Modes & Actions
Vietnamese – Pain Response & Respect for Authority

Preservation/Maintenance
- Respect for elderly and those in authority
- Family support
- Education and working hard

Accommodation/Negotiation
- Time management
- Health practices
- Communication style ~ eye contact
- Conflict resolution

Repatterning/Restructuring
- Extend knowledge about other cultures' responses to pain

Resources

Capell, J., Dean, E., Veenstra, G. (2008). The relationship between cultural competence and ethnocentrism of health cae professionals. *Journal of Transcultural Nursing.* (19)2, 121-125.

Calvillo, E. R., Flaskerud, J. H. (1991). Review of literature on culture and pain of adults with focus on Mexican-Americans. *Journal of Transcultural Nursing.* (2)2, 16-23.

Douglas, M. (1999). Pain as the fifth vital sign: Will cultural variations be considered? *Journal of Transcultural Nursing.* (10)4, 285.

Nowak, T. T. (2005). Vietnamese. In Lipson, J. G., Dibble, S. L., (Eds.) Culture & Clinical Care. San Francisco CA: UCSF Nursing Press.

Hunter, J. L. (2008). Applying constructivism to nursing education in cultural competence. *Journal of Transcultural Nursing.* (19)4, 354-362.

Kavanagh, K. H. (2008). Transcultural perspectives in mental health nursing. In Andrews, M. M., Boyle, J. S. (Eds) *Transcultural Concepts in Nursing.* (5th Ed.) Philadelphia, PA: Lippincott Williams & Wilkins

Leung, P.K., Boehnlein, J. (2005). Vietnamese Families. In McGoldrick, M., Giordano, J. Garcia-Preto, N. (Eds) *Ethnicity & Family Therapy.* (3rd Ed.). New York: Guilford Press

Leininger, M. M. (1997). Understanding cultural pain for improved health care. *Journal of Transcultural Nursing.* (9)1. 32-35.

Leininger, M. M. (1991). Culture care diversity and universality: A theory of nursing. New York: National League for Nursing Press.

Leininger, M. M., McFarland, M. R. (2002). Transcultural nursing: Concepts, theories, research and practice. (3rd Ed.). New York: McGraw-Hill.

Lovering, S. (2006). Cultural attitudes and beliefs about pain. *Journal of Transcultural Nursing.* (17)4, 389-395.

Ludwig, P (2008). Transcultural aspects of pain. In Andrews, M. M., Boyle , J. S. (Eds.) Transcultural Concepts in Nursing Care. (5th Ed.). Philadelphia: Lippincott Williams & Wilkins.

Peters, M. (2000). Does constructivist epistemology have a place in nursing education. *Journal of Nursing Education.* (39)4, 166-172.

Purnell, L. (2008). People of Vietnamese Heritage. In Purnell, L.D., Paulanka, B.J., (Eds.) *Transcultural Health Care: A Culturally Competent Approach.* (3rd Ed.). Philadelphia, PA: F.A. Davis Company

Ramer, L., Richardson, J. L., Cohen, M. Z., Bedney, C., Danley, K. L., Judge, E. A. (1999). Multimeasure pain assessment in an ethnically diverse group of patients with cancer. *Journal of Transcultural Nursing.* (10)2, 94-101.

Spector, R. (2009). *Cultural diversity in health and illness.* (7th Ed.), New Jersey: Pearson/Prentice Hall.

Stauffer, R. Y. (2008). Vietnameses. In Giger, J. N. Davidhizar , R. E. (Eds.) Transcultural Nursing: Assessment and Intervention. (5th Ed.). St Louis, MO: Mosby/Elsevier.

Wisneski, L. A., Anderson, L. (2005). The Scientific Basis of Integrative Medicine. New York: CRC Press.

Yoder, M. (1997). The consequences of generic approach to teaching nursing in a multicultural world. *Journal of Nursing Education.* 35, 315-321.

Yoder, M. (2001). The bridging approach: Effective strategies for teaching ethnically diverse nursing students. *Journal of Transcultural Nursing.* 12, 319-325.

Don't Touch My Wife . . . Someone Call for Assistance!

(Arab Muslim)

18

Herman Maldanaldo steps back, anger flickering in his eyes   He is not a diminutive man, 5'10" and counting, but his medical practice at Elmwood Emergency has kept him slim and wiry – that and the jogging each morning before he comes in. Omar Masmoudi, however, is intimidating.

Mr. Masmoudi is not unlike the doctor with olive complexion or height, but he seems to be empowered by demons, ferocious ones, when it pertains to his wife Benizar.

"You will not touch her," he says.

Mrs. Masmoudi is groaning, gurgling as she gasps for air.

Dr. Maldanaldo advances towards the patient, intent on ignoring her husband as he performs his ER duties. Omar bars the way. He is grieving for Sasha, his young sister-in-law, who was just learning to drive when the truck swerved into her lane so near the exit for home. But he is mainly focused on his wife.

"You will NOT touch her."

The Masmoudi family, Omar, Benizar, and their son Sunni, have lived in Fremont for six years now. Surrounded by Arabs from most of the countries in the Middle East, they feel amazingly secure in this foreign land. Everyone they know keeps agreements and respects elders, whether Afghani, Pakistani, or Moroccan. They are bound together by the Qur'an, the holy book. In their neighborhood it has not seemed unusual for someone to excuse himself for a gathering to pray. No one drinks alcohol, except for a few of the men in their twenties, but they will come to their senses; it is only for effect as they toy with the idea of pursuing seductive Western girls. Good Muslim women, of course, will not let anyone other than another woman touch them in public.

So what is this doctor thinking? Omar has told him to keep away from Benizir. Her accident is making him more distressed than his wife seems to be. She is moaning a little, but an examination by this imbecile is not what she needs. What she needs is to find balance, balance between choler and phlegm perhaps. The car crash has upset her system, not just her head; the gash over her left eyebrow is only a symptom. And now this doctor fellow keeps trying to get her to look at him in the eye. How incredibly rude. If there were a woman doctor on duty, he would consent to an examination, but this Maldanaldo fellow is just too insensitive, to unaware of propriety.

"You will not touch my wife."

Herman Maldonaldo feels his hands tighten into fists. This man is impossible. How is he supposed to examine Mrs. Masoudi if her loud and swaggering husband does not get out of the way?

"Before the water reaches the bridge," begins Omar, but the doctor, focused on treating his patient, ignores him. He calls to a nurse to bring Security, immediately.

"This woman may die if I can not examine her to assess the extent of her injuries. I will not be barred from doing what good I can, even if her husband has different ideas.

Understanding the tension . . .

The Qur'an provides the structure and guidelines to follow for gender roles and modesty. Women are not to be touched by someone other than their husband. We can readily understand the frustration of Mr. Masoudi when a male physician presents to examine his wife. However, as we often see in the emergency room when time is of the essence, care for the patient may supersede religious dictates. Unless the situation is life threatening, is there another way to resolve this dilemma other than escorting Mr. Masoudi out of the room? Written policies and procedures that address issues of modesty and gender roles help establish protocol and avoid confrontations. Unspoken here is the voice of Mrs. Masoudi. Might she feel the same anxiety as her husband? Our responsibility is to provide care in a respectful and expedient manner. How well we do this well is dependent on our knowledge of the patient's religious beliefs and values, along with flexibility to deliver care.

The tenets . . . the beliefs held true to faith

The Qur'an, the holy book of Islamic faith, is believed to be the literal word of God. It furnishes guidelines for all aspects of one's life. Transmitted by the Angel Gabriel to the prophet Muhammad in the 7th century AD, the Qur'an is considered absolute truth and outlines the norms for social allegiance and behavior. The word Islam translated means *submission to Allah* (God), or the act of *submission*, or *resignation to God*, or *submits to the will of God*, depending on the source. Each aspect or situation in life is the will of Allah. The Hadith (tradition) is the sayings and deed of the prophet Muhammad. Recognition of sharia law by Muslims includes the five sections of human behavior: required, encouraged, permissible, discouraged and prohibited (Andrews, Hanson 2004).

The division of Muslim people into Sunni and Shi'ite occurred following the death of Muhammad. Some felt that the next leader should be decided by an electoral process, while others strongly believed that a descendant should hold the leadership position. These two groups emerged: Sunni (electoral) and Shi'ite (descendent). Both subscribe to the principles and practices of the Islamic faith and the Qur'an. There are five basic pillars of Islam that guide each person.

Five Pillars of Islam

- Testimony of the unity of God and prophethood of Muhammad (Shahadatan)
- Prayer five times a day (salah)
- Almsgiving and social responsibility to the poor (zakah)
- Fasting during the month of Ramadan (sawm)
- Performance of the pilgrimage to Mecca, the Hajj

Hammad et al. (1999 p.13)

Reflective exercise: Incorporating the practices

1. *Is there a policy that addresses issues of modesty and gender roles in the Arab Muslim?*
2. *Is there a policy to ensure the patient's ability to meet the obligations of prayer five times each day?*
3. *What policies are in place regarding "difficult visitors"? Does it take into consideration cultural beliefs, values, and obligations?*
4. *Are there prayer areas in your facility that can be used by family members?*
5. *What are some other aspects about the Islamic faith that you would like to know?*
6. *Where do you find common ground?*

Culture consistent with history

One cannot understand the Muslim culture without some knowledge of history. Emigration from the Middle East to the United States began in the late 1800s with people seeking economic opportunities. Reasons for the second, third, and fourth waves of immigration resulted from the political and social upheavals in the Middle East. Following relaxation of immigration laws in 1965, a significant number of persons reunited with their families in the United States.

Their cultural beliefs, values, and practices sustain them in times of transition to a new place, as well as with management of healthcare issues, disability, and death. As HCPs we need to consider the Muslim American's culture and the tenets of Islam that are woven throughout the patient, family, and community. Research from studies done in the Detroit area of Michigan, which is said to have the largest Arab Muslim population in the United States (Luna 1989, Leininger 1991), and other areas of the country help us to understand the caring practices of this community.

Arab Muslim Cultural Values & Beliefs

1. Follow the teachings of the Qur'an
2. Responsibility for providing care and support to family
3. Respect gender roles and responsibilities
4. Modesty
5. Offering respect and privacy for religious practices
6. Obligation and responsibility to visit the sick
7. Helping to save face and preserve cultural values

Each provide a foundation from which the patient derives support and assurance that care given is in accordance with guidelines provided in the Qur'an. In our vignette, three aspects are highlighted: modesty, gender, and family responsibility. Mr. Masoudi, husband and patriarch, is an advocate for his wife, ensuring that she receives care that is consistent with their beliefs. Women and men may not interact socially outside of the extended family, and modesty in dress is essential; hence, the importance of same-sex providers in the clinical setting. As mentioned earlier, this can be suspended in a life-threatening situation, yet it is best to have a contingency plan in place to avoid potential conflict. Mr. Masoudi has the obligation to be his wife's advocate and to remain with her. Dr. Maldonaldo has the obligation to provide emergency medical care. The emergency room staff has the obligation to be knowledgeable about the cultural beliefs, values, and health practices of the Muslim patient.

Reflective exercise: Cultural ways of being
1. *How are your cultural values and beliefs different from Arab Muslims?*
2. *Where do you find common ground?*
3. *How do you accommodate family members?*
4. *What are some creative innovations that could have been used?*

Family affair . . .

It is sometimes said, "if the Qur'an is the soul of Islam, then the family can be described as the body." As with other ethnic groups, the individual sees himself within the context of the unit. Family always comes first. The tradition of patriarchy and hierarchy is the structure from which family obligations emanate. Young give deference to the elderly, and women are subordinate to men. The gender roles are seen as complementary, each serving a purpose that contributes to the well-being and ongoing support of the family. Extended family, those related by blood, and women who joined through marriage provides socioeconomic and social support.

The husband is the main economic provider, protector, and decision maker. In an extended family, the eldest male may assume the decision-making role. Women are responsible for the maintenance of the home, healthcare, education, and child rearing. Modesty is an important value held by the Muslim woman. Clothing permissible for family events is different from that worn in public. The covering of body except for the face and hands is thought to provide protection. Wearing the *hijab* (head covering) outside is a symbol that indicates her status as a Muslim and her desire to send that message to all who see her. For HCPs, it heightens awareness of the importance placed on modesty, especially during a physical examination. Acknowledgment communicates respect for her cultural and religious practices.

Children are highly valued and loved. They are taught, at an early age, the values of loyalty, duty, obligation, and respect for their parents and elders. Close family ties are maintained throughout their lifetime. Discipline is usually meted out by the father. The mother serves as an intermediary during difficult times. Sacrifices are made to ensure educational opportunities. How well the child does academically and socially is a direct reflection on the family.

Elderly are honored and shown respect at all times. With age comes status and self-esteem, especially for women. Elders are thought to be wise and provide counsel to the younger generation. They should be addressed formally, using the title and first name. Responsibility of elder care falls to the adult children, usually the eldest son. It is expected that the elder will live with the son until death. Nursing homes would not be considered appropriate.

Communication

In the vignette, Mr. Masoudi appears loud, intrusive, and demanding. There are two important issues to recognize in this situation. First is the importance of modesty for his wife and, second, that he is the patriarch and the voice of his family. It is within his role to assert himself. We are not given the details of his wife's condition, but if Mr. Masoudi knew the gravity of the situation, he might allow the physician to proceed.

Think about a time when a family member was in the emergency room. You, as a HCP, wanted to be the voice, the advocate, for that person. You may have thought "I am a professional health person therefore entitled or obligated to speak up." This might have led to a misunderstanding between you and the physician and staff. While these are different circumstances, it helps us to understand the urgency and anxiety felt by Mr. Masoudi that led to his outburst and eventual eviction from the room.

Communicating loudly and quickly, for the Arab Muslim man, means that the message is important. It is repeated until the recipient comprehends the urgency. Body language is expressive and conveys the importance of the message as well. It may seem aggressive to an outsider, but normative for the Arab Muslim culture. Women may seem reserved and passive, showing little expression in the clinical setting. It is important to note that nodding may not infer agreement or understanding, but rather politeness and avoidance of disagreement.

Eye contact and touch are defined along gender roles. Both are valued in conversation between male communicants. Women avoid eye contact with men and strangers. Touch is limited to same gender. Handshakes do not occur between genders. Allow the patient to extend a hand first before extending your own. The value of same gender HCP provides a comfortable encounter that corresponds with the values, beliefs, and practices of the Arab Muslim patient.

Creating a welcoming environment that includes time for informal discussion prior to the exam can make a world of difference in the outcome.

Time . . .

Past and present orientations are important to the Muslim patient. Past includes adherence to and belief in the Qur'an; following rituals such as prayer and making a pilgrimage are valued. In present orientation, social events are loosely scheduled according to the importance of the event and not the time participants arrive. However, business interactions are timely.

The strong value placed on reliance on the will of Allah does not negate health promotion or prevention practices. According to Yosef (2008) the teachings of the Prophet Mohammed encourages one to stay healthy and to seek care if needed. If one does not know what is written for the future, participation in preventative health programs may indeed be part of what is written. Making assertions about what may or may not occur in the future is not consistent with the belief in the will of God. For example, if the HCP indicates that at some future date an illness will resolve, the Muslim patient may add, In sha Allah – God willing.

Health Beliefs

In sha Allah "if God wills" is the cornerstone of belief that God predetermines all events and situations, including health and illness. Cancer may be seen as a result of Divine Will and not due to a behavior such as smoking. It is out of the control of the individual and implies that everything good and everything bad is the result of God's actions.

The value of healthcare in Islam is based on the belief that "God created human beings and gave them their bodies as gifts to be cared for. On the Day of Judgment, God will ask what they did with their bodies and their health" (Yosef 2008 p.287). There is an obligation to care for one's self by following the teachings in the Qur'an related to prayer, diet, hygiene, and exercise. One may not seek professional healthcare first, but rather seek the advice of family. Establishment of relationship and rapport with the patient is enhanced when family is included. Information is more forthcoming once trust is part of the equation.

In addition to God's will or punishment, cause of illness for the Muslim patient may be due to other reasons. Physical illness can be caused by an imbalance of the hot and cold/dry and moist elements found in the Four Humors (Chapter 9). Home remedies are used to restore balance. The patient/family's perception of the condition will dictate the treatment. It is important for the HCP to inquire what treatments were used prior to the appointment and to discuss the effectiveness of the remedy. Wind may also have an adverse affect on the health of an individual, thus procedures such as cupping and moxibustion (Chapter 9) may be used.

Two values highlighted in the vignette, modesty and gender roles, are important to acknowledge in the clinical setting. The Islamic concept of aura is defined as those parts of a woman's body that should never be seen by an unrelated member of the opposite sex. Only the hands and face can be exposed. During an appointment, the Muslim woman may appear passive in conversation and action, especially if the provider is male. Exposing part of the body may instill a feeling of guilt or shame for not following the teaching of the Qur'an. In a study done by Kulwicki et al. (2000), one patient stated, "it's like ayb (shame) to talk about this (women's health issues) with a male doctor." Allowing a female relative to be present during an exam may provide assurance.

Mental illness comes with a social stigma, as is common for many cultural groups. The patient may present with various somatic complaints. Privacy about family matters may also keep the individual from seeking care in the early stages. The Muslim patient may be considered touched by an evil spirit or demon, or seen as receiving a punishment from Allah. Supernatural causes of illness can be averted by wearing amulets and turquoise pendants and by wearing verses from the Qur'an. In the case of children, protection is provided by invoking Allah when complimenting a child.

221

Patience, perseverance, and suffering are valued responses to illness, because it is Allah's will, and the purpose does not need to be known by the patient.

The hospitalized patient. . .

Caring for an ill person is the obligation of family and extended family. The patient takes the passive role during illness. In the hospital setting, family members remain present and assist in the care. While it may seem an intrusion for the staff, it is an opportune moment to learn from family about those caring practices that promote recovery. Collaboration by HCPs demonstrates a genuine interest. Visitation by extended family is expected by the patient. Prayers and recitations from the Qur'an for healing may be a communal activity.

Observing and performing prayer five times each day is important to maintain health and prevent illness. It is done before sunrise, noon, midday, sundown, and nighttime. Washing of the mouth, nose, face, ears, back of neck, hands, and arms up to the elbows prior to recitation of prayers ensures purification. The patient may ask "which way is east" and hopefully the HCP will have that answer. Accommodating the patient with this valued ritual instills appreciation that the HCP is aware of and sensitive to their spiritual needs. Fasting, during the month of Ramadan may pose a dilemma for the patient. Unless health issues are significant, the fast includes abstinence from food, drink, and medications from before sunrise until after sunset. Discussion with an elder or an Imam from the Mosque may convince the person that fasting is not required given the health status of the patient.

Detary needs are to be taken into consideration, too, including avoiding all pork products and the requirement that meat be properly slaughtered (halal). It is important to note that some processed foods may contain animal fat and thus should be avoided as well. The patient may follow a vegetarian diet during the stay or may have family bring food from home.

Death and sharing bad news

What if Mrs. Masoudi dies? Illness and death, like other events, happen according to Allah's will. It does not negate the value of life or mean that grief is any less than that found in other ethnic groups. It is an extremely difficult time, emotionally and physically. For many, their religious faith and practices provide assurance and support during this process. Death in the Muslim faith is considered the ending of this life and the entering of the afterlife for judgment.

For the gravely ill patient, prolonging life or life support may not be deemed appropriate if there is little hope of recovery. Discussion of death is avoided, however. For a HCP to talk about an impending death may be seen as interfering with the will of Allah, and it could be perceived as the cause of an earlier death.

When counseling family members about their loved one it is important to ask, "who is the spokesperson?" This individual is responsible for informing the family.

Following death, extended family and community members may arrive at the hospital and remain with the person until transport. An Imam from the Mosque may recite passages from the Qur'an. Expression of grief comes after the death and not before. It may be loud, vocal, and seem uncontrolled. "Wailing and gasping is a common reaction in grieving" (Hammad et al. 1999 p.24).

Autopsy is seen as a mutilation of the body and will be strongly opposed. Reaction by family members to a request from the HCP for an autopsy may be hostile. A request for organ donation may be met with a similar response, as it is important that the body remain whole. Acculturation and knowledge about the benefits of organ donation may help them to be open to this request. All conversations should be done respectfully with the understanding and acceptance that the family may refuse.

*   *   *   *

The Arab Muslim patient provides us, as HCPs, with a unique perspective on life and the influence of Islam religion on healthcare practices. The challenge for the HCP is to understand, accept, and incorporate many of these cultural values and beliefs into the plan of care. Understanding the hierarchal structure, defined gender roles, and the importance of extended family helps to assure that the HCP is aware of each of these when caring for the patient. Acknowledgment and respect lead to rapport and trust between patient and HCP.

Culture Care Modes & Actions
Arab Muslim – Emergency Situations

Preservation/Maintenance
- Hierarchical family structure
- Modesty and gender roles
- Prayer five times each day

Accommodation/Negotiation
- Dietary needs
- Minimal eye contact and touch ~ women
- Extended family
- Folk practices
- Religious beliefs

Repatterning/Restructuring
- Provider preference in life threatening events

Resources

Abdel-Halim, A. (2008). Did you know? Refuting rigid interpretations concerning the position of women in Islam, and Muslims' interactions with non Muslims. Northmead, NSW: Akbar's Print Management.

Abudabbeh, N. (2005). Arab Families. In McGoldrick, M., Giordano, J. Garcia-Preto, N. (Eds) *Ethnicity & Family Therapy*. (3rd Ed.). New York: Guilford Press

Al-Omari, H., Scheibmeir, M. (2009). Arab Americans' acculturation and tobacco smoking. *Journal of Transcultural Nursing*. (20)2, 227-233.

Andrews, M. M., Hanson, P. A. (2008). Religion, culture and nursing. In Andrews, M. M., Boyle, J. S. (Eds.) Transcultural Concepts in Nursing. (5th Ed.). New York: Lippincott Williams & Wilkins

Galanti, G. A. (2004). Caring for Patients from Different Cultures. (3rd Ed.). Philadelphia: University of Pennsylvania Press.

Hammad, A., Kysia, R., Rabah, R., Hassoun, R., Connelly, M. (1999). Guide to Arab Culture: Health Care Delivery to the Arab American Community. MI: ACCESS Community Health Center, Health Research Unit.

Islamic Council of Queensland. (1996). Health Care Providers Handbook on Muslim Patients. Australia: Queensland Health.

Kulwicki, A. D. (2003). People of Arab Heritage. In Purnell, L. D., Paulanka, B. J. (Eds.) Transcultural Health Care: A Culturally Competent Approach. (2nd Ed.). Philadelphia: F.A. Davis.

Kulwicki, A. D. (2008). People of Arab Heritage. In Purnell, L. D., Paulanka, B. J. (Eds.) Transcultural Health Care: A Culturally Competent Approach. (3rd Ed.). Philadelphia: F.A. Davis.

Lawrence, P., Rozmus, C. (2001). Culturally sensitive care of the Muslim patient. *Journal of Transcultural Nursing*. (12)3, 228-233.

Leininger, M. M. (1991). Culture care diversity and universality: A theory of nursing. New York: National League for Nursing Press.

Leininger, M. M., McFarland, M. R. (2002). Transcultural nursing: Concepts, theories, research and practice. (3rd Ed.). New York: McGraw-Hill.

Luna, L. J. (1989). Transcultural nursing care of Arab Muslims. *Journal of Transcultural Nursing*. (1)1, 22-26.

Meleis, A. I. (2005). Arabs. In Lipson, J.G., Dibble, S. L., (8th Ed). Culture & Clinical Care. San Francisco CA: UCSF Nursing Press.

Shusta, R. M., Levine, D. R., Wong, H. Z., Olson, A. T., Harris, P. R. (2008). Multicultural Law Enforcement: Strategies for Peacekeeping in a Diverse Society. (4th Ed.) New Jersey: Pearson, Prentice Hall.

Simpson, J. L., Carter, K. (2008). Muslim women's experiences with health care providers in a rural area of the United States. *Journal of Transcultural Nursing*. (19)1, 16-23.

Spector, R. (2009). *Cultural diversity in health and illness*. (7th Ed.), New Jersey: Pearson/Prentice Hall.

Yosef, A. R. O. (2008). Health beliefs, practice, and priorities for health care of Arab Muslims in the United States. *Journal of Transcultural Nursing*. (19)3, 284-291.

Just Say No . . . But To Whom?

(Chinese)

19

"Maybe it's just the change of life," Anita thought. "I think my mother stopped her monthlies early too. I'm tired all the time, too tired to flirt with that cute Lewis Eng even. Too much moon energy's going on, I guess."

Anita and Lewis were two of the techie friends from UC Berkeley who had started Quicklink. There were five of them, always a difficult number, but it had turned out to be helpful for breaking ties when there were differences of opinion. Henry usually took the opposite view from Lewis. Anita sided with her boyfriend almost always, and Cynthia and Sharon were the swing votes. All that didn't matter much at the moment, of course, since Quicklink had abruptly dissolved due to the recession.

"I don't want to have to move to the South Bay. Even if Lewis found a job nearby, it's awfully far from the whole Ling family. Girls aren't expected to be successful, I know, but if I don't have children I'd like to do something I enjoy."

Anita yawned as she tipped her brass watering can carefully into the Ming-style pot where her prized Christmas cactus grew. Recently she'd felt as prickly as her plant, unable to find a comfortable position in bed much less sleep. And when Lewis had asked her to dinner at Henry's Hunan last week for a consolation dinner, Anita could hardly taste her favorite roast duck. Not that she'd had much appetite recently.

Won Ling, Anita's father, had given her a bagful of huang qi formula from the store, and she'd tried to take it religiously. That first night she had slept better or at least she thought so. But ever since her symptoms had persisted. Since the demise of Quicklink, while looking for another job and finding only a couple of leads in Saratoga, she'd scheduled an appointment at the Pacific Avenue Clinic too. Anita liked Ashley, her nurse practitioner. Ashley Johann was about forty also, but looked a lot younger with her long blond hair and white teeth.

"I bet she hasn't even thought about the change," Anita sighed. "And I bet she'll be angry about my father's herbs too. Maybe I'll just avoid the whole confrontation by canceling Tuesday. I certainly won't be able to look her in the eye if I have to mention huang qi, but I'd have to, wouldn't I?"

*   *   *   *

Beliefs and value . . . when they don't match

Cultural beliefs and values are so ingrained in who we say we are that Anita feels caught between the respect for her father's remedies and the potential reaction by her nurse practitioner. She may not want to question or disagree with the treatment provided by either; however, the dilemma is whose treatment plan to follow. A third generation Chinese American, Anita's outward appearance portrays her as being very American in her conversation and style of dress. She had been successful, socially and economically. Now, the loss of the start up company, her creative group of friends at Quicklink, and minimal prospects for employment have left a void in her life. This disharmony Anita feels is an indicator for her that something, physically, emotionally, or spiritually, is wrong. Deciding what to do about it can cause even more tension, considering the values and beliefs of the Chinese American cultural group.

Chinese Culture Values & Beliefs
- Harmony and unity
- Compliance and respect for those in authority and the elderly
- Family loyalty
- Communal assistance
- Folk practices and treatment modes
- Importance of hard work and giving to society

Harmony and balance are important values in the Chinese culture. Respect and honor for those who are elderly and those in authority provide harmony through the hierarchal structure. Family loyalty provides support when crisis or illness occurs.

Communal assistance is consistent with the belief that the group is more important than the individual. This teamwork approach, similar to Anita's experience at Quicklink, shows respect for each member. Those in leadership positions have a responsibility to consider the interests of the worker, and workers count on that person to ensure their needs are met.

Reflective exercise: **Harmony and balance . . .**
1. *Where do you find harmony and balance in your life?*
2. *Are families involved in the health care of their members?*
3. *How are your values and beliefs different from the Chinese American?*
4. *Do you notice a difference between first generation and second generation Chinese Americans?*

Historically speaking

The importance of working hard and as a group dates back thousands of years in the Chinese culture. This value helped the Chinese people to endure hardships, specifically the famine that followed the Opium Wars of 1830 with England and 1856 with France. As a result of the famine, many emigrated to the United States in the mid 1800s. They were well received and appreciated. Work was abundant and gold plentiful. However, as the economics in America began to change, animosity toward the Chinese immigrant increased. As immigrants, they were barred from becoming citizens. They had no civil rights under the law. Racial prejudice and violence were common especially during this economic downturn. The Chinese, working for low wages, were seen as "taking all the jobs away from Americans."

The 1882 Chinese Exclusion Act was the first immigrant law passed that targeted a specific group of people. The law excluded all Chinese laborers from coming into the country and restricted those currently in the United States from traveling between the two countries. Deciding to return to China meant they would not be allowed to return to the U.S., thus making it virtually impossible to provide for their families. The law was repealed with the passage of the Magnuson Act of 1943.

Between 1910 and 1940 Angel Island, located in the San Francisco Bay, was the processing center for Chinese immigrants. Some of these immigrants wrote poetry and signed their names on the walls of the barracks. Angel Island has been recently restored and is now considered a historical site. Many people come from around the country to see where their ancestors arrived as immigrants.

Today, Chinese Americans, who number 2.5 million, make up the largest group of Asian Americans in the United States and, according the the U.S. Census Bureau (2008), are the third largest immigrant group after Mexicans and Filipinos. Also, Chinese is the most widely spoken "other language" following Spanish. While most Chinese Americans reside in California or New York, the demographics are beginning to change.

Family – hierarchy and generations

Family and extended family are highly valued. Two or three generations may live in the same household. Value is centered on the concepts of togetherness, unity and harmony. This collectivistic approach provides assurance for support financially, physically, and emotionally. Commitment to family supersedes personal needs. During times of illness, each member of the family participates in the care of the individual. This responsibility may cause family members to change their work schedules or living arrangements in order to care for others until recovery is assured.

Hierarchy and patriarchy continue to be part of the structure of family and extended family. Clearly delineated roles and responsibilities help ensure harmony within the family, with the youngest showing deference and respect to the elderly and those in authority. Decisions, which may include consultations with other members of the family, are expressed by the father or the eldest son. Women, in addition to possibly working outside the home, are the primary caregivers of the children and the elderly parents.

Children are held in high value and are expected to do well in school. Academic achievement reflects positively on the parents' child-raising skills. In addition, a good education is believed to lead to socioeconomic stability, ensuring the adult child's ability to care for their aged parents and to pay for the funeral expenses.

The elderly are held in high esteem by family and community. Today many care for the grandchildren, rather than sending them to a daycare center. They are the keepers of the wisdom and tradition. They may live with the eldest son rather than in a nursing home. An Asian American pharmaceutical representative shared with me that, "Of course I wouldn't put my mother in a nursing home because she is 'experiencing her second childhood' and I will be there to care for her during that time."

> **Reflective exercise: Family . . . then and now**
> 1. *Are your patients traditional Chinese, Acculturated Chinese, or a combination of both?*
> 2. *In what ways is your family of origin different from the traditional Chinese family?*
> 3. *How are the families involved in the healthcare of their members?*
> 4. *Where do you find common ground?*

Communication

Hoping to win the coveted "Civilized City" award, Guangzhou, China, is trying to clean up its city. There are three requests made of the Chinese people. First, no spitting; second, tone down the loud conversation, especially around tourists; and third, when standing in line don't push. Spitting is common in China. Why do people spit? The answer is twofold: it is a result of smog and pollution and because "we've always spit." Pushing while in line is said to be from times of famine when people had to stand in long lines waiting for food (Foreman 2009).

Chinese are expressive and may seem loud to outsiders. The conversation is fast and usually very animated. Non verbal communication, commonly used within the family, is reserved around outsiders. Eye contact is considered rude and disrespectful and used sparingly. Minimal eye contact, especially with the elderly, shows the value placed on harmony and hierarchy. Responding with a nod and smile or verbally saying yes may really mean no. As HCPs we must consider this type of response and inquire further before deciding on a plan of care. Silence is valued; allow time for patients to make decisions. In addition, touch should be kept at a minimum.

Recently, an elderly Chinese woman presented at our clinic. She had fallen during a tour at a local winery. She spoke no English so her adult daughter interpreted for her. As a Certified Transcultural Nurse, I sought to recall the Chinese cultural beliefs, values and appropriate procedure to follow: The head is considered sacred and the feet unclean. I knew that if I examined the leg first, it would be inappropriate to return to the upper torso, so I began the examination taking her vital signs and listening to her heart and lungs. At the conclusion of the exam, she bowed to me. I thought "okay" and I bowed back. She bowed. Finally, after about three reciprocal bows, she stopped. I did appreciate the opportunity to practice my transcultural skills. It made the appointment meaningful for me and hopefully for her too.

Time

The owner of a hotel destroyed during the tsunami in Indonesia in 2006 and now being rebuilt was asked by an international television journalist if the tourists were returning. His response, "Well the Brits and the Americans aren't coming because they are afraid of another tsunami, and the Asians are not come back because of the ghosts." They are very different reasons, yet each is valid to that particular cultural group. In the Chinese culture, the sudden and unexpected death of an individual is believed to cause their spirit to become a menacing ghost, that is until a special ceremony is held to placate the spirit. In the book, *Snow Flower and the Secret Fan*, by Lisa See, a young girl Beautiful Moon is stung by a bee and dies.

> Everyone knows that part of the spirit descends to the
> afterworld while part of it remains with the family . . . The
> way Beautiful Moons unhappiness came to us every night in
> Aunt's otherwordly moans let Snow Flower and I know we
> were in danger. Snow Flower came up with a plan. "A flower
> tower must be made," she said one morning. A flower tower
> was exactly what was needed to appease Beautiful Moon's
> spirit.
>
> See 2003 p. 98

The past is still present in the Chinese culture. Ancestors are part of the family. They offer protection and guidance to those left behind. An annual event called Sweeping the Tomb, similar to El Dia de los Muertos in the Mexican tradition, is held in the fall and the spring. Families show respect to the ancestors by tending their gravesites and celebrating their lives by telling stories.

Time, thought of as circular in nature, allows the past and future to be intertwined with the present moment. One may not seek healthcare unless symptoms cause a disruption with the flow of daily activities. This may conflict with the HCP's view of time that emphasizes prompt response to health concerns. As noted before, future orientation for the Chinese American patient focuses on the value of education. Both education and respect for the elderly help to assure the parents that the adult child will have the means to care for them.

> <u>Reflective exercise</u>: Past . . . Present . . . Future
> 1. *Is it an expectation that you care for your elderly parents?*
> 2. *And pay for their funerals?*
> 3. *Does your family have rituals to honor ancestors?*

Health practices

Although Anita is third generation acculturated Chinese American, she values treatments that may not align with the western medicine. Many patients are reluctant to discuss alternative treatments used prior to coming to their appointment. This hesitancy may stem from a distrust of the system or possibly from past encounters with HCP that have not gone well. One cannot assume that if a patient appears very "American," like Anita, that cultural beliefs and health practices are not valued.

At a seminar on cultural awareness education that I provided for a large medical facility, a young Chinese American nurse shared his story. He was in college, and had just been diagnosed with diabetes. His mother and grandmother insisted that he try their mixture of herbs and chicken body parts before he started the medication prescribed by his HCP. He shared with us that, out of respect for his mother and

232

grandmother, he would follow their herbal treatment for two weeks. He "knew" it would not work, but then there was a piece of him that believed that maybe, just maybe, it would be effective.

It's all about balance and harmony in body, mind, and spirit. The principle of Chinese medicine, *Yin* and *Yang*, embraces that concept. These two opposing yet complementary forces are found in every aspect of the universe. *Yin* is female, dark, cold, and creator of the earth; while *Yang* is male, lighter, hot, and creator of the heavens. Health and well-being occur when there is balance; illness comes with imbalance. Eating specific foods designated as either *Yin* or *Yang* aid in the recovery because each offers a restorative balance. Maintaining good relationships with family and others also helps to maintain harmony and avoid illness. Treatments include acupuncture when there is excessive *Yang* and moxibustion (cupping, coining and leeches ~ see Chapter 9) when there is excessive *Yin*. Various herbs are used to restore balance, also.

Chi, also known as *qi*, is the term for energy and is found in all living things. It is kept in balance by the *Yin* and *Yang*. It circulates throughout the body to provide nourishment and to eliminate bad *qi*. The channels through which it flows are all interconnected; thus, if there is an imbalance in one area, another area may be affected. Acupuncture (a cold treatment) is a Chinese practice that is used when there is excessive *Yang* in the body. The procedure includes an inspection of the patient's physical appearance, tongue, and palpation of pulses. A variety of needles, each with a specific purpose, are inserted into particular points along the meridian (pathways of *qi* flow) in the body. This technique restores balance, thus curing disease and relieving discomfort or pain.

Treatment from a Chinese herbalist may be sought when, after consulting family and friends, an illness persists. One only needs to venture down to Chinatown in any thriving metropolitan area to find an herbalist who offers remedies for a given condition. In the book by Amy Tam, *Bonesetter's Daughter* (2001), the protagonist's father was an herbalist. Tam describes many of the herbs that were used by families living in China at the time, and continue to be used today.

Anita thinks that, although she did experience relief the first night, the results from the herbs were less than she expected. From her perspective, the symptoms may be due to menopause. Anita's symptoms of fatigue and a decreased interest to socialize might lead her HCP to a different diagnosis. It might be helpful to consider other possibilities for her imbalance of *Yin* and *Yang*. Is she going through menopause, or is she depressed? A patient may present with somatic complaints such as fatigue, insomnia, and headache. These symptoms provide a socially acceptable way to address a problem and avoid any discussion of mental illness. In the Chinese culture, mental illness comes with a negative stigma.

Our protagonist is uncomfortable sharing this information with her father or her nurse practitioner. Avoidance of conflict and confrontation is an important value held in the Chinese culture. Anita wants to improve her current health situation, but as we can see from the story, harmony and balance seem to elude her.

The stigma of mental illness does not allow for acknowledgment of symptoms, therapy sessions, or pharmaceuticals. How do we approach the subject in a nonintrusive manner? One way is to focus on the symptoms. Open-ended questions that promote discussion may help to show the patient a correlation. Here are some initial inquiries that might be helpful to process the information:

> **Reflective exercise: Questions for Anita . . .**
> 1. *What makes you think this might be menopause . . . how do you feel about that?*
> 2. *When did these symptoms begin?*
> 3. *What do you think caused them to start when they did?*
> 4. *What have you tried to help alleviate them . . . food . . . herbs . . . exercise?*
> 5. *Have these treatments been helpful?*
> 6. *Was there some significant event that occurred at the same time?*

Each encounter provides an opportunity for the HCP to gain the trust and respect of the patient, which is especially important when emotional or mental issues are involved. As we gain knowledge about alternative therapies, Yin and Yang food, herbal teas, and exercise programs commonly used by the Chinese patient, we can engage in the discussion more fully.

An interesting study caught my eye while doing research for this chapter. The author Yi-Kue Tsai (2009) suggested that I Chin Ching (Muscle/Tendon exercises), a style of ancient Chinese qugong and similar to t'ai chi, improves circulation and qi as well as increases muscle strength and endurance. This exercise is thought beneficial if initiated prior to and throughout the course of menopause. Slow and simple movements are coordinated with inhalations and exhalations. Believing that this form of exercise is easy to learn, Tsai posited that the beneficial effects of increased circulation and qi would also help prevent osteoporosis and heart disease. The results: increased muscle endurance. Being knowledgeable about styles of exercise such as Tai Chi and I Chin Ching may afford HCPs a broader perspective of treatment options.

Religious beliefs and practices

Think about those times when spirituality or religion influenced your perception about an illness, a disability, or an injury. Did it give you the strength or insight to deal with the uncertainty?

Chinese Americans may embrace several spiritual practices: Buddhism, Confucianism, Taoism, Shamanism, and Christianity. The teachings of Buddhism and Taoism have shaped the values found in the Chinese culture and include harmony, respect for life, and the balance of the Yin and Yang. These lead to a practice of simplicity, patience, humility, and avoidance of conflict. Confucianism focuses on the hierarchical roles that clearly define relationships and respect for those who are elderly and in authority. Health and well-being derive from keeping balance in one's life, in relationships with others, and with the environment. We are not told to which belief system that Anita subscribes, but we do see her loyalty to her father and her desire to avoid conflict with her nurse practitioner. As you care for Chinese American patients, think of ways that their religion and spiritual practices can be incorporated into the plan of care.

*   *   *   *

Anita's hesitancy to talk with her nurse practitioner may be due to previous encounters, or possibly to stories heard from other family members and relatives who experienced opposition to herbal treatment. As we understand more about the culture, we help to assure good health outcomes and trusting relationships.

Culture Care Modes & Actions
Chinese – Herbal Therapy & Acculturation

Preservation/Maintenance
- Respect for elderly and those in authority
- Family loyalty
- Communal support

Accommodation/Negotiation
- Folk treatments and practices
- Minimal eye contact
- Avoidance of conflict

Repatterning/Restructuring
- High expectations leading to increased stress
- Collaboration with HCP

235

Resources

Andrews, M. M. (2008). The influence of cultural and health belief systems on health care practices. In Andrews, M. M., Boyle, J. S. (Eds.) Transcultural Concepts in Nursing Care. (5th Ed.). New York: Lippincott Williams & Wilkins.

Chen, Y. H., Caine, R. M., Wang, M. F. (2009). Depression in Chinese immigrants. Advance for Nurse Practitioners. May. 35-40.

Chin, P. (2005). Chinese. In Lipson, J. G., Dibble, S. L., (8th Ed). Culture & Clinical Care. San Francisco CA: UCSF Nursing Press.

Foreman, W. (2009). Gritting city polishes image to satisfy Beijing. *San Francisco Chronricle*. August 30, 2009.

Galanti, G. A. (2004). Caring for Patients from Different Cultures. (3rd Ed.). Philadelphia: University of Pennsylvania Press.

Gladwell, M. (2008). Outliers: The Story of Success. New York: Little, Brown and Company.

Hall, L., Callister, L. C., Berry, J. A., Matsumura, G. (2007). Meanings of menopause: Cultural influences on perception and management of menopause. *Journal of Holistic Nursing*. (25)2, 106-118.

Im, E. O., Chee, W. (2005). A descriptive internet survey on menopausal symptoms: Five ethnic groups of Asian American university faculty and staff. *Journal of Transcultural Nursing*. (16)2, 126-135.

Lee, E. Mock, M. R.. (2005). Chinese Families. In McGoldrick, M., Giordano, J. Garcia-Preto, N. (Eds) *Ethnicity & Family Therapy*. (3rd Ed.). New York: Guilford Press

Leininger, M. M. (1991). Culture care diversity and universality: A theory of nursing. New York: National League for Nursing Press.

Leininger, M. M., McFarland, M. R. (2002). Transcultural nursing: Concepts, theories, research and practice. (3rd Ed.). New York: McGraw-Hill.

Lloyd, K. B., Hornsby, L. B. (2009). Complementary and alternative medications for women's health issues. *Nutrition in Clinical Practice*. (24)5, 589-608.

Ma, G. X., Du, C. (2000). Cultually competent home health service delivery for Asian Americans. *Home Health Care Manager Practices*. (12)5, 16-24.

See, L. (2003). *Snow Flower and the Secret Fan*. New York: Random House.

Spector, R.. (2009). Cultural diversity in health and illness. (7th Ed) New Jersey: Pearson/Prentice Hall.

Tam, A. (2001). The Bonesetter's Daughter. New York: The Ballantine Publishing Group.

Tsai, Y. K., Chen, H. H., Lin, I. H., Yeh, M. L. (2009). Qigong Improving physical status in middle-aged women. *Western Journal of Nursing Research*. (30)8, 915-927.

U.S. Census Bureau. (2008). Facts for Features: Asian/Pacific American Heritage Month. 1-8. Wang, Y. (2003). People of Chinese Heritage. In Purnell, L. D., Paulanka, B. J. (Eds.) Transcultural Health Care: A Culturally Competent Approach. (2nd Ed.). Philadelphia: F.A. Davis.

Wang, Y., Purnell, L. (2008). People of Chinese Heritage. In Purnell, L. D., Paulanka, B. J. (Eds.) Transcultural Health Care: A Culturally Competent Approach. (3rd Ed.). Philadelphia: F.A. Davis.

Willgerodt, M. A., Killien, M. G. (2004). Family nursing research with Asian families. *Journal of Family Nursing*. (10)2, 149-172.

Wisneski, L. A., Anderson, L. (2005). The Scientific Basis of Integrative Medicine. New York: CRC Press.

Xu, Y., Chang, K. (2008). Chinese Americans. In Giger, J. N., Davidhizar, R. E. (Eds.) Transcultural Nursing: Assessments and Interventions. (5th Ed.). St Louis, MO: Mosby/Elsevier.

Oh That Youthful Image . . . Where Did It Go?

(Anglo)

20

Staying forever . . . Young

Cindy comes out of the daze slowly, her mouth dry, her fingers clammy. All she can think of is that quote . . . from Drew Cary? . . . about high school reunions. She'd just seen it in the pink section of the Chronicle, the scrambler puzzle page, about how there are only six months to make ourselves perfect when reunions come to mind. She readjusts the wire feeding into her left arm so that it covers a liver spot she'd found last week.

"How can I have a liver spot when I'm not even finished with my period yet? Damn. I wonder if Tammy has any; I bet not. She'll be there for sure at Novato High. She was runner up class president, wasn't she?"

Cindy is not a complainer. She adjusts another wire over a freckle. Her sandy blond hair show just a hint of gray, but she hopes no one will notice they'll be so impressed with her svelte figure. Which is not that shapely any more actually, but Cindy knows that it will be. What did Drew Carey say? Six months? She'll just stop eating bread and potatoes and cake and ice cream and pizza and . . . And of course the gym. She can go after work.

As she becomes more alert she wonders, "What are these tubes anyway? I have to get going," Cindy muses. "At least I'm a big success at Valtech, won salesperson of the year award last fall, didn't I? If only Frankie and Melinda could see that instead of my flabby butt. Did anyone call my office or get in touch with Ashley to say that I won't be at her soccer game? What time is it anyway? I have to get going."

Cindy's family members were all achievers. Her great-grandfather had been a teamster for UPS at the turn of the century, when teamster really meant team of horses. He'd come over from Ireland at the end of the Gold Rush in California.

239

Like all of his ancestors and descendants, he seemed to relish hard work. He'd driven a team of Morgans from dawn until dusk until his death at 43. Great-grandma Rose has raised the seven kids by herself then, managing to send them all except Uncle Fred to the university. She'd taken in sewing and taught school and helped Dr. Pratt with his book work, never complaining.

So what is Cindy doing now? She can't feel sorry for herself. Her body just isn't cooperating, but she'd fix that! A tear slides quietly down her left check into the pillow, but Cindy will not sniff, she will ignore it, just as she'd ignored her hypertension. Her family was strong.

"Maybe I'll dye my hair," she thinks.

*   *   *   *

Individualism, competition, and achievement are values that were established early in Cindy's life and continue to influence her present day decisions and actions. This country's history, from the perspective of the Anglo American person, begins in the mid 1600s with the establishment of Jamestown on the eastern seaboard. The puritans (they preferred to call themselves separatist), were portrayed as hard working individualists who fled England for a better life. They worked industriously and tirelessly to ensure success. These themes of individualism and separatism carried into the late 1700s when they declared themselves independent from English rule with the writing of the Declaration of Independence.

The 1880s were a time of westward movement – a "pioneering spirit" was the theme. Railroads were built to increase migration from east to west. The Gold Rush of 1848 also drew many to the west. This era exacted a cost to individuals and families, but the values of working hard and achieving success far exceeded the complacency of staying in place.

As Americans moved west, a large contingency of emigrants came from Europe seeking a better life, willing to work hard to achieve the "American dream."

Cindy's values are aligned to those who came before her and set the stage for her life as well.

Cultural Beliefs and Values

Let's look at the values and beliefs of the Anglo American culture, which Dr. Leininger describes in her ethnostudies as white, middle and upper class persons. Individualism and self-determination are recurring themes that emerge from her and other researcher's studies.

Anglo Cultural Values & Beliefs

- Individualism
- Independence and freedom
- Competition and achievement
- Instant time and actions
- Youth and beauty
- Egalitarian
- Reliance on scientific facts and numbers
- Earned respect for authority and the elderly
- Generosity in times of crisis.

Leininger et al. 1991 p. 355

Similarly, in 1949 Kluckhohn describes the American national character as an individualistic, self-reliant, high achieving, yourth-oriented, benevolent optimist who believes in equality and freedom. He goes on to say that this individualism is explained by activities and achievements and that the consequences, good or bad, are taken personally (Spangler 1991). It is interesting to note that in one-fourth of all Americans descended from English colonists, even with intermarriage with other ethnic groups, the Anglo American core values remain dominant in these families (McGill, Pearce 2003).

Reflective exercise: Perspective . . .
1. *From your perspective, do these values reflect American culture?*
2. *Are these values and beliefs found in other cultural groups?*
3. *Are individualism, self-reliance, and competition found at your health institution?*
4. *Do you think those values benefit and motivate staff?*
5. *How are your cultural beliefs and values different?*
6. *Where do you find common ground?*

Communication

Communication is how we reveal ourselves to others . . . a reflection of our cultural beliefs, values, and ways of living in this world. We develop our style from our family of origin and later from peers and colleagues. How we share information is personal and at the same time cultural. The aspects of effective communication listed here are important, especially if one wants to "do well" in a professional career.

241

Valued Communication Elements

- Good eye contact
- Firm and strong handshake
- Name it and say it
- Get to the point

Expressing oneself, while maintaining an emotionally controlled response, shows an inner strength and reserve. Conversation is linear and the focus is on getting to the point quickly and concisely. Extended dialogue, "meaningless meandering" as they see it, is thought to waste the listener's time. Words are chosen carefully to articulate a clear message. Loud and fast describes the communication style. The tone of voice usually reflects the meaning of the message. There is an expectation of eye contact during a conversation. This may be in direct conflict with some cultural groups who consider eye contact rude and disrespectful. While a handshake is welcomed from outsiders, touch is reserved for those within the circle of friends and family. Communication in the social setting may be the same or more relaxed in all aspects.

> **Reflective exercise: Communication as heard and observed . . .**
> 1. *How is your style different from the Anglo American?*
> 2. *Where do you find common ground?*
> 3. *Do your patients have a similar style?*
> 4. *How would you need to modify your approach to meet the needs of a patient with the style of communication listed here?*

Time . . . is of the essence

Time is money. Plan for the future. These are two adages that are synonymous with the time orientation for the Anglo American. Future time orientation holds the most importance and aligns well with the values of self-reliance and individual achievement. Dwelling on past events is seen as a distraction to planning for the future. Schedules are viewed as a necessary and organized way to deal with multiple events, ensuring that nothing is left to chance. The message is that time is of the essence and is not to be wasted. This time orientation may cause conflict with colleagues in the workplace. The Anglo American's future orientation relies on setting priorities, organizing tasks, and getting work done in a timely manner. Those who are present oriented are more attentive to the "here and now." This may cause tensions between colleagues.

Future planning, as in "saving for a rainy day," secures future needs such as money for college education or retirement. One colleague stated that, even though she hated her job, "If she just worked three more years full time instead of her current part time status, she'd be able to retire with more money."

In our vignette, Cindy is planning for that reunion (future orientation) and she wants to look like she did many years before (past orientation). She has difficulty focusing on the present. As HCPs we can acknowledge her goal to "look good like I used to" for the upcoming event, but also help her see that her current activities are having a negative effect on her health. Designing a program that is realistic and acceptable to her is the challenge.

For those who value future consideration, conflict can occur when opposing views are presented. Acknowledging the differences can bring about a willingness to collaborate on a plan of care. That is the hope we have with Cindy.

So what about conflict . . .

Conflict. Avoid it at all cost or face it head on. How one defines what is a problem and how it should be resolved varies. When stressed, individuals generally rely on behaviors and attitudes that evolved from their cultural roots. The Anglo American values of autonomy and self-reliance translate to adages such as "stand up for oneself" and "confront the perceived injustice." The ability to maintain a distant and stoic stance while forming a logical response is held in high esteem. One who avoids conflict may be viewed as weak. The stronger the belief that one's perspective is correct, the more escalated the conversation may become. In the clinical area, coming on too strong with an opinion may have a negative impact on relationships with colleagues and patients.

<u>Reflective exercise</u>: **The best way to deal with conflict is . . .**
1. *Avoid it?*
2. *Face it?*
3. *Tell someone else about it?*
4. *Ask someone to be your intermediary?*
5. *How are you the same or different from your colleagues or patients?*

Families

In our opening vignette, there is no mention of family or friends. Cindy may hold the belief that she can handle the situation and support is unnecessary. Anglo American families distinguish themselves from other ethnic groups with the emphasis placed on the individual and not the group. Individual freedom and self-determination provides the foundation with which to pursue life's ambitions. The results of a study done by McGoldrick (2005) with American mental healthcare professionals found they were raised in families in which "men and women were expected to be independent, strong, and able to make it alone . . . self-control was highly valued" (p. 437). Dependence on others, especially those outside of the family, was seen as weakness.

Family structure is shifting from the traditional nuclear family, defined as a married man and woman with a child, to blended families, single parent families, same sex, and communal families. An egalitarian structure does not preclude an imbalance at home. Many women have a professional career and mange family responsibilities. They may present to the clinic with a variety of health concerns that seem to relate fatigue, mentally and physically. This may also be seen with some men who are assuming the childcare responsibility and working. It is important that we as HCPs not assume family roles and responsibilities, but inquire of our patients about their current family structure and support system. As families relocate to various parts of the country, support may come from colleagues, friends, or religious and social organizations.

While today's families are seen as egalitarian, decision making in high-income families may be patriarchal. At our seminars we pose this question: "Who was the decision maker in your family of origin?" followed by "Who is it in your current family?" Many respondents state it was their father, but in their current family structure it is egalitarian. Herein may lie the conflict. What if you value autonomy and an egalitarian approach to decision making and your patient, an Arab Muslim woman, values patriarchy and relies on her husband to make all the decisions. Where do you find common ground?

Health beliefs

Individualism, achievement, youth orientation, reliance on facts, and the value of time are aspects that must be considered when planning for healthcare of the Anglo American patients. These values and beliefs influence the decision to seek care and guide the patient's healthcare practices. For Cindy, the desire to achieve her goal to lose twenty pounds and look like she did twenty years ago supersedes her interest in health maintenance. She would not be in the emergency room hooked up to monitors or intravenous lines had she not subscribed to the belief that she could "do it all." While this may seem like an exaggeration, we have only to view ads on television or in magazines to understand the value placed on youth. As HCPs we are not called to judge, but to understand that one's cultural beliefs and values influence healthcare practices.

The Anglo American view of healthcare is predominately focused on a western or a biomedicine approach: cause and effect. Illness is caused by a virus, bacteria, poor diet, lack of exercise, exposure to toxins and yes, on occasion, stress. Patients may present with a list of questions as well as information they have found through friends or on the internet. If the HCP is unable to provide the care they hoped for then a referral to a specialist, or better yet, the "best known physician" in the field is expected. For those in the middle and upper socioeconomic level, the reliance on facts to determine how an illness should be treated is essential. Facts provide the assurance that the right diagnosis is made and the best treatment plan is initiated.

Today there is a move toward a naturalistic or homeopathic view of health and wellness. The use of herbal teas and medicines, acupuncture, and yoga has increased over the past years. Some insurance companies are now covering alternative forms of therapy. A recent television news story highlighted the therapeutic use of Reiki, a method used to increase energy in the body, following chemotherapy. The results showed that the procedure alleviated symptoms of nausea and fatigue. Herbal teas and drugs, such as Black Cohosh, are effective in the treatment of menopausal hot flashes. Saw palmetto is used by men to help prevent prostate cancer. These are self-reports. Little research has been done on herbal medicine to validate its effectiveness. It is important for the HCP to be aware of and discuss with the patient the potential interactions and side effects of all of their medicines, including over-the-counter (OTC) drugs and herbal remedies.

An increased awareness and acceptance of nutrition and exercise are important elements to consider in physical and mental wellbeing. During an annual exam, the HCP can discuss the patient's normal eating habits and physical exercise. With the availability of gyms and exercise centers, more people are participating in exercise programs. A new concept called extreme sports (parasailing off cliffs) has entered into the vocabulary and lives of many Anglo Americans. It aligns well with the values of hyperindividualism and competitiveness. Yet it is not without risk physically and mentally.

Another newly diagnosed condition, primarily found in the Anglo American group, is called exercise bulimia. It is found mainly in young women who start a healthy exercise regime and then begin to use it compulsively to control their weight. It almost cost the life of one woman. In a television interview, she shared that she exercised three hours each day, seven days a week. Interestingly, though, during the interview she stated that, "I had more health problems during that time than I ever had before." So the values of competition, self reliance, and individualism can be seen as both beneficial and potentially harmful to the patient.

Our job as HCPs, as with all patients, is to develop a trusting relationship. Once established, the patient may share more information about health concerns, use of herbal and OTC drugs, nutritional habits, and exercise regimes. While our patient Cindy is already planning her future from the emergency room cubicle, it is imperative that we as HCPs acknowledge her world view. It may not match ours, but we can find common ground to provide her with care and health education that meets her needs.

If we view her as an individual, understand her value of self reliance, and allow her to be part of the decision-making process in the plan of care, it helps ensure compliance.

<u>**Reflective exercise**</u>: **Caring for those who value self-reliance . . .**
1. *What are the challenges you face caring for the Anglo American patient?*
2. *Does your facility provide information on extreme sports?*
3. *What alternative therapies are available at your institution?*
4. *How are your views different from those of your Anglo American patients?*
5. *Where do you find common ground?*

* * * *

Developing a plan of care that considers the health issues in combination with the patient's cultural beliefs and values requires that we find ways to build a foundation based on those concepts. Cindy has spent a lifetime with the values of independence, self-reliance, and competition. They have served her well. She is successful in her business ventures, which brings positive accolades from her colleagues and family. She has an image to protect, and it appears that in our vignette, she is determined to succeed regardless of future consequences. She has future goals, and we as HCPs can provide her with information about future outcomes if she continues with her current plan. We start where she is at this moment, listen, acknowledge her story, and provide guidance toward a healthy lifestyle.

Culture Care Modes & Actions
Anglo – Health Maintenance

Preservation/Maintenance
- Independence
- Acknowledge and face conflicts
- Competition

Accommodation/Negotiation
- Communication style
- Exercise regime

Repatterning/Restructuring
- Nutritional intake
- Prescription medication regime
- Work/Life balance
- Present timeline for reunion

Resources

Andrews, M. M., Boyle, J. S. (2008). Transcultural concepts in nursing care. (5th Ed.).New York: Lippincott Williams & Wilkins.

Banks, J. A., McGee-Banks, C. A. (2004). Multicultural Education: Issues and Perspectives. (5th Ed.). New Jersey: John Wiley & Sons, Inc.

Cronin, B. (2001). Knowledge management, organizational culture and Anglo-American higher education. *Journal of Information Science.* (27)3, 129-137.

Edelman, D., Christian, A., Mosca, L. (2009). Association of acculturation status with beliefs, behaviors, and perceptions related to cardiovascular disease prevention among racial and ethnic minorities. *Journal of Transcultural Nursing.* (20)3, 278-285.

Galanti, G. A. (2004). Caring for Patients from Differenct Cultures. (3rd Ed.). Philadelphia: University of Pennsylvania Press.

Giger, J. N., Davidhizar, R. E. (2008). Transcultural nursing: Assessment and intervention. (5th Ed.).St Louis, MO: Mosby/Elsevier.

Giordano, J., McGoldrick, M. (2005). Families of European Origin: An Overview. In McGoldrick, M., Giordano, J., Garcia-Preto, N (Eds.) *Ethnicity & Family Therapy.* (3rd Ed.). New York: The Guilford Press.

Juarbe, T. C., Lipson, J. G., Turok, X. (2003). Physical activity beliefs, behaviors, and cardiovascular fitness of Mexican immigrant women. *Journal of Transcultural Nursing.* (14)2, 108-116.

Leininger, M. M. (1991). Culture care diversity and universality: A theory of nursing. New York: National League for Nursing Press.

Leininger, M. M., McFarland, M. R. (2002). Transcultural nursing: Concepts, theories, research and practice. (3rd Ed.). New York: McGraw-Hill.

McGill, D. W., Pearce, J. K.. (2005). AmericanFamilies with English Ancestors from the Colonial Era: Anglo American. In McGoldrick, M., Giordano, J. Garcia-Preto, N. (Eds) *Ethnicity & Family Therapy.* (3rd Ed.). New York: Guilford Press

Purnell, L. D., Paulanka, B. J. (2008). Transcultural Health Care: A Culturally Competent Approach. (3rd Ed.). Philadelphia, PA: F. A. Davis Company.

Sellers, S. C., Poduska, M. D., Propp, L. H., White, S. I. (1999). The health care meanings, values and practices of Anglo-American males in the rural Midwest. *Journal of Transcultural Nursing.* (10)4, 320-

330.
Shusta, R. M., Levine, D. R., Wong, H. Z., Olson, A. T., Harris, P. R. (2008). Multicultural Law Enforcement: Strategies for Peacekeeping in a Diverse Society. (4th Ed.) New Jersey: Pearson, Prentice Hall.
Spangler, Z. (1991). Culture care of Philippine and Anglo-Saxon nurses in a hospital context. In Leininger, M. M., McFarland, M. R (Eds.) Culture Care Diversity & Universality: A Theory of Nursing. New York: National League of Nursing Press.
Spector, R.. (2009). Cultural diversity in health and illness. (7th Ed) New Jersey: Pearson/Prentice Hall.

Blueprint For Success . . .
Planning Care That Fits With
& Is Beneficial To Whom?

21

"From the patient's perspective"

A *blueprint* sounds so simple. Yet, the final outcome is dependent on participants having a clear understanding of the project and a willingness to work together to make it a success. In the healthcare field, success comes when the HCP and the patient are in agreement about the plan of care. Both have a stake in the outcome. Quality care and culturally competent care are key elements that provide the foundation.

Each successful encounter between the HCP and the patient builds a trusting and respectful relationship in which both have the ability to agree, disagree, and ultimately find common ground. The blueprint begins with the acknowledgment that cultural beliefs, values, and health practices of the HCP (western medicine) may contrast with the patient's (folk practices). When the patient's healthcare practices include both, biomedicine and folk, there is common ground from which to begin a dialog. Demonstrating a keen interest and openness to another's perspective promotes collaboration. Each encounter with the patient can further establish rapport, respect and trust.

In this chapter, we walk with a patient from the front door of a clinical setting to various encounters with staff. We identify elements that promote understanding of cultural differences and recognize aspects that help to create a welcoming environment.

Walking through the front door . . .
Consider a patient and family walking through the front door of your institution. What do they see first? An information desk? A greeter? How do they know where to go? Are signs written in a language that they

understand? They may think, "Is there anyone here who looks like me or speaks my language?" While each of these components may seem small, for the patient it may make all the difference. Health institutions can be overwhelming to a person who already feels ill and anxious. In the blueprint for success, the first message to patients is "all are welcome," with the subtitle, "there are no barriers here." Cultural awareness, sensitivity, and competency begin at the front door and continue with every encounter:

> **Reflective exercise**: A welcoming environment
> 1. *In what way does your institution send the message "you are welcome here"?*
> 2. *Do you see any barriers that might send another message?*
> 3. *Is the mission statement visible?*
> 4. *What languages are spoken and by whom?*
> 5. *Are staff, professional and ancillary, reflective of the community?*
> 6. *What would you add to make it even more welcoming?*

Signing Consents . . . important aspects to consider

There are many forms for the patient to read and understand, including consent for admission/treatment, release of information, advanced directives, and of course the financial responsibility and privacy forms. You are familiar with these forms – several pages, small print, single space. A request to read and sign them may seem daunting. It is reported that most consent and admission forms are written at the college level, while most signers are at the fifth grade level. This can be an intimidating task for a person with minimal education and/or limited English proficiency. Not wanting to seem ignorant or waste the clerk's time, patients sign the form without knowing what they have just signed. Can you imagine how much time it would take if the patient actually read the entire form?

From a cultural perspective, this is an opportunity to ask the patient if there is someone else who should be involved in this process. In many cultural groups, the head of the family is the one to read the form first. In addition, consideration can be given to simplifying the form and making it available in the patient's language. These simple changes build on the foundation to create a welcoming place.

Imaging – Lab draws – Procedures . . . and Cultural Influences

Procedures such as blood draws, x-rays, medical imagining, and other nonsurgical treatments, may be considered intrusive by some patients.

Cultural beliefs may cause some patients to hesitate or delay these diagnostic procedures. For example, some Chinese, Hmong, and Vietnamese believe that drawing too much blood may weaken the body, causing heat to be lost, thus making them more vulnerable to illness. Acknowledging this belief prior to the procedure, and allowing for discussion of fears, may alleviate the anxiety of the patient.

For some cultural groups such as the Native American population, having an x-ray or a MRI may equate to being photographed. A belief is held that a soul can be lost when a picture is taken. This may preclude compliance with a request for such a procedure. Knowledge of various beliefs and open discussion with patients prior to procedures sends a message of openness and understanding.

Here are some questions the HCP can ask: . . .
1. Offer explanation of the consent or procedure.
2. Allow time for questions.
3. Acknowledge cultural beliefs and health practices.
4. Listen to the verbal and observe the nonverbal response of the patient ~ do they match?

If admitted to the hospital . . . who decides?

Who makes healthcare-related decisions varies from culture to culture and from generation to generation. A first generation Chinese-American may subscribe to a patriarchal belief – the father or the eldest son is the decision maker. A fourth generation Chinese-American, more acculturated to the Western lifestyle, may espouse an egalitarian or individualistic belief. In the Cuban culture, the most educated, most respected, eldest family member, male or female, is consulted. The Native American culture, which may vary from kinship to kinship, values autonomy. One does not speak for another, though one's decision is tempered by the effect it may have on family and community. Decision making in the Mexican, Hmong and Southeast Asian cultures may involve family members and the extended family. While there seems to be a patriarchal predominance in many cultural groups, education, acculturation, and socioeconomic status are changing that norm.

How can the HCP know which group adheres to which belief and practice? The key to a successful encounter comes with knowledge and experience. When the HCP does not know, then some questions to ask the patient are as follows: "How are decisions made in your family?" and "Who is involved in that process?" and "Is consultation with a family member necessary prior signing a consent form for a procedure, a treatment or a surgical procedure?" Asking these questions lets the patient know that you have an interest in knowing and continues to build a foundation of trust.

> **Reflective exercise**: **Decision-making/Spokesperson**
> 1. *How were decisions made in your family of origin?*
> 2. *Is that different from your family of today?*
> 3. *How is your decision-making mode different from that of your patients?*
> 4. *Where do you find common ground?*

The Importance of Families

Our family of origin shaped our world view, instilled beliefs, and implanted the value of family. For many, family is the foundation and support to which one looks during times of illness. How that impacts the operations of a healthcare organization can translate into a negative or positive experience.

My initiation into the field of cultural care came when the physical therapy department at a local hospital requested an inservice for staff. It seems the problem centered, not on the staff, but rather on their Mexican American patients' failure to return for follow-up appointments. In their words, these patients were noncompliant. Unfortunately, from the perspective of some HCPs, the term noncompliance invokes a negative image of patients who are either irresponsible or unconcerned for their health. A second issue raised by the staff was that when the patient did show, the entire family came as well. It created, as one staff person said, an "inconvenience for staff" due to limited space. From the patients' perspective, this was not a welcoming place, thus they did not follow up with care.

The inservice focused on the cultural beliefs, values, and healthcare practices of the Mexican American patient, specifically the importance of family support. The staff gained an insight. This paradigm shift created an eagerness on the part of the staff to create an environment that welcomed families. The increase in compliance to follow up with their appointments led to healthier outcomes and increased both staff and patient satisfaction. Think about the patients served by your organization. In what ways are families included and welcomed to participate?

Reflective exercise: How do you include family members?
1. *In outpatient settings?*
2. *During procedures or treatments?*
3. *In the emergency room?*
4. *In the Intensive Care Unit?*
5. *In the Pediatric Unit?*
6. *In the Obstetrical Unit?*
7. *During end-of-life?*

Oh, those visitors . . .

For many groups visiting the hospitalized patient is highly valued and obligatory. For staff, visitors may be viewed as intrusive and affect their ability to "get the work done" by the end of the shift. While it can be overwhelming to have twenty to thirty persons in the waiting room, creating a venue for visitation may actually improve the health and well-being of the patient. An integral part of the blueprint for success occurs when the HCP acknowledges that "family is everything" for many cultural groups.

Consider the ill patient and the impact of the illness on family. What is the role of the sick person? For many cultures (Mexican, Filipino, Chinese, Roma and others), the ill person takes on a passive role, enabling and expecting family members to provide care. However, in the dominant culture of the U.S., value is placed on self-reliance. Although appreciating offers of help during their infirmity, these individuals are more likely to want to manage on their own.

Could this create difficulty for the HCP who promotes independence by encouraging the patient to do for him or herself? From the perspective of the HCP self-care ensures a successful recovery, but it may be in direct conflict with a patient's belief of family participation during illness. Taking the opportunity to collaborate with family sends the message of respect for differences and willingness to find common ground. It is a blueprint for success.

Reflective exercise: Role of the Sick Person
1. *What was the role of the sick person in your family of origin?*
2. *How is it different from that of your patients and their families?*
3. *Where do you find common ground?*
4. *In what ways do you encourage the patient's family to participate in the patient's care?*

Influences of Cultural Health Beliefs and Practices . . .

Chapter 9, *Ancient Wisdom . . . Modern Medicine*, gives a view of cultural healthcare practices from three perspectives: biomedicine, personalistic, and naturalistic. Each one offers insight into the cause and the cure of illnesses. For some, the cause is bacteria, for others an angry ancestor, still others an imbalance of Yin and Yang. What if these beliefs impact recovery? How can the HCP acknowledge those beliefs?

Dr. Leininger's three modes and actions, discussed in Chapter 7, address the benefits and concerns of each perspective. Culture care maintenance and/or preservation, culture care accommodation and/or negotiation, and culture care repatterning and/or restructuring serve as guides for the HCP to consider when developing a plan of care. The more aligned patients are with their culture, the stronger the belief in its efficacy. As we review each decision-making mode, think about your clinical experiences. Was there a "disconnect" between you and the patient/family? Was there something you could have done differently?

Culture Care Preservation/Maintenance

From a patient's perspective, these beliefs and practices may mean the difference between recovery or relapse. Support by preserving and maintaining beneficial health beliefs can be shown by incorporation of these practices into a plan of care. For example, wearing protective amulets such as crosses (Mexican, Filipino), star of David (Jewish) or strings around the wrist (Hmong) serve as protection against illness and provide an inner sense of wellbeing.

I had the occasion to do a home health visit to a pregnant Mexican-American woman. She was on bedrest due to an episode of premature labor the month prior. Upon entering the home, I noticed an altar on a nearby table. A candle and a religious card depicting the Virgin of Guadalupe, protector of mothers and infants, were displayed. Acknowledging this in our discussion assured her that I understood the value placed on her beliefs. Recognizing those beliefs increases rapport and promotes trust.

Culture Care Accommodation/Negotiation

Are there times when we need to negotiate with or accommodate our patients? Yes, and flexibility is the key to success. Does this health practice provide a sense of hope and well-being for the patient, and can it be negotiated into the plan of care? It may seem small to us, but the effect for the patient will be huge. Our acceptance of their belief sends a clear message to the patient that we are listening and are willing to negotiate, accommodate, and incorporate these components into the plan of care.

Some examples of cultural care accommodation/negotiation include flexibility with family and when they accompany a patient to an appointment or procedure. Some cultural groups consider it an obligation and duty to visit the hospitalized patient or to spend the night with the patient in a hospital setting. This help to ensure a feeling of comfort, safety, and security for the patient. Family members wishing to provide care during a hospitalization may seem counter-productive to our encouragement of "self-care," but negotiating a dualistic approach, and providing an understanding of why, can be a win-win situation for all.

Preserving language is another method that fosters acceptance by our patient. If you have ever traveled to a foreign country and did not speak the language, you can understand how difficult it must be for our patients to express themselves in English. As we know, the ability to speak one's own language provides more information about their illness and the increases acceptance of a treatment plan. Bilingual, bicultural healthcare professionals provide that bridge to understanding. It sends the message that the organization acknowledges the needs of the non-English speaking people.

Cultural Care Repatterning/Restructuring

What if those cultural beliefs, values, and healthcare practices of the patient are, from the HCP's perspective, harmful? What then? Education, open discussion and collaboration with the patient and family can make a difference in outcomes. These are strongly held beliefs; thus, to repattern takes time. It requires attentiveness to the patient's current beliefs and, through a respectful interchange, brings about an awareness of the negative effect this belief may have on his or her well-being.

Restructuring a patient's dietary pattern when diabetes has been diagnosed may seem like an uphill struggle. For example, a diabetic patient with uncontrolled blood sugars as a result of dietary intake can face long-term consequences. Creative ways to restructure dietary and exercise patterns may involve patient, family and community. On a recent trip to the southwest, we visited the city of Tuba, Arizona. It is home to the Hopi Indians. The grocery store we entered had a table that showed food that was acceptable for diabetics. Written in the native language as well as in English, the sign exhibited the amount of calories, fat, carbohydrates, and protein for each item. It was visually appealing, causing us (outsiders) to pause and review the display. As a HCP, I was impressed to see the innovative way this information was shared in this community.

Balancing beliefs . . .

Balancing beliefs . . . Providing Quality Care (Figure 21-1) displays elements that must be considered when planning care that is beneficial to the patient and family. It is a balancing act: each component must be addressed. When health professionals and organizations are knowledgeable about their own cultural beliefs, values, and health practices and those of their patients, then culturally competent and quality care is assured. Respect and knowledge completes the picture. It is a blueprint for success.

> **Reflective exercise: From your perspective . . .**
> 1. *Where is it difficult to provide balance between patient and HCP?*
> 2. *Which element would pose the greatest obstacle?*
> 3. *How would you incorporate cultural beliefs and practices into a plan of care?*

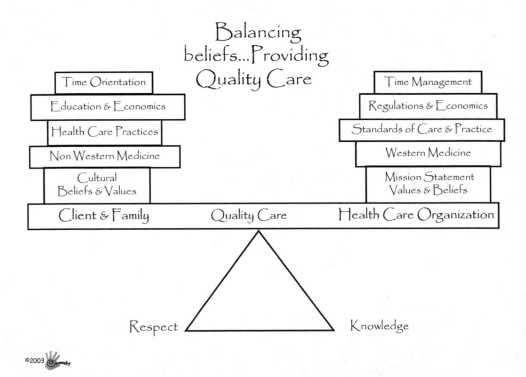

Figure 21-1: Balancing Beliefs . . . Providing Quality Care

Patient Education ~ When It Works Well

We Learn
10% of what we see
20% of what we hear
30% of what we read
50% of what we see, hear, and read
70% of what we discuss with others
80% of what we experience
90% of what we teach

Dr. William Glasser & Dale Eager

The chart, originally designed by Dale Eager in the 1950s with the onset of television, and then later modified by Dr. William Glasser, provides an insight into how one learns, given the mode. In other words, by reading this book you would retain about 30%. Look what happens though when you take that information and discuss it with a colleague: you remember 70%. With an actual experience you remember 80%. Now think about your patient population. Which of the modes would be the most effective for them? Each educational opportunity is unique. Results are contingent upon additional variables such as age, educational level, language, and literacy.

So how can we make it meaningful for the patient? The first, and simplest, approach is to ask the patient, "how do you learn best?" Begin at that point and then assess the effectiveness of that method. Is the patient able to provide a return demonstration or reiterate information received during a video or lecture? A clear understanding of the information promotes self assurance for the patient and confirmation for the HCP that patient understands the material.

Staff Education ~ When It Makes Caring Effective

Why cultural awareness education for staff? HCPs who have attended our seminars state that they were excited about putting into practice all that they have learned. It sparked a desire in them to collaborate with patients, families, and colleagues. In addition, having the knowledge motivated them to develop standards of care and practice, policies, and procedures that address culturally competent care.

Educational opportunities come in a variety of formats, such as periodicals, journals, seminars, and experiences. Case presentations are one of the best ways to convey information about cultural health practices and beliefs. These can include a multidisciplinary team and persons from the community. Following the presentation, HCPs leave with a broader, holistic view of health, wellness, and healing that can be incorporated into future encounters.

*   *   *   *

A blueprint for success includes a willingness on the part of the staff and the healthcare facility to participate in creating a welcoming environment for the diverse ethnic populations they serve. Understanding that cultural beliefs, values, and health practices are unique to each patient and family challenges us in the healthcare field to embrace diversity to help ensure positive outcomes for those seeking care. Openness to new experiences broadens our perspective and elightens us in unexpected ways.

Resources

Andrews, M. M., Boyle, J. S. (2008). Transcultural concepts in nursing care. (5th Ed.). New York: Lippincott Williams & Wilkins.

Campinha-Bacote, J. (2003). The process of cultural competence in the delivery of healthcare services: A culturally competent model of care. Cincinnati, OH: Transcultural C.A.R.E. Associates.

Dale, E. (1969). Audiovisual Methods in Teaching. New York: Drained Press: Holt, Rinehart and Winston.

Gay, G. (2000). Culturally responsive teaching: Theory, research & practice. New York: Teachers College Press.

Giger, J. N., Davidhizar, R. E. (2008). Transcultural nursing: Assessment and intervention. (5th Ed.). St Louis, MO: Mosby/Elsevier.

Joint Commission on Accreditation of Healthcare Organizations. (2004). Standards, intents and examples for patient and family education and responsibilities.

Jones, P. S., Zhang, X. E., Siegel, K. J., Meleiss, A. I. (2002). Caregiving between two cultures: An integrative experience. *Journal of Transcultural Nursing*. 13(3), 202-209.

Leininger, M. M. (1991). Culture care diversity and universality: A theory of nursing. New York: National League for Nursing Press.

Leininger, M. M., McFarland, M. R. (2002). Transcultural nursing: Concepts, theories, research and practice. (3rd Ed.). New York: McGraw-Hill.

Lipson, J. G., Dibble, S. O. (2005). Culture & Clinical Care. San Francisco CA: UCSF Nursing Press.

McGoldrick, M, Giordano, J., Garcia-Preto, N. (2005). *Ethnicity & Family Therapy*. (3rd Ed.). New York: Guilford Press

Menghini, K. G. (2005). Designing and evaluating parent educational materials. Advances in Neonatal Care. 5(5), 273-83.

Purnell, L. D., Paulanka, B. J. (2008). Transcultural Health Care: A Culturally Competent Approach. (3rd Ed.). Philadelphia, PA: F. A. Davis Company.

Sandoval, V. A., Adams, S. H. (2001). Subtle skills for building rapport using neuro-linguistic programming in the interview room. *FBI Law Enforcement Bulletin* 1-5.

Spector, R.. (2009). Cultural diversity in health and illness. (7th Ed) New Jersey: Pearson/Prentice Hall.

Vandervort, E. B., Melkus, G. (2003). Linguistic services in ambulatory care. *Journal of Transcultural Nursing*. (14)4, 358-366.

Cultural Competence in Healthcare Organizations . . . Who Cares?

22

Health disparities, defined by the American Academy of Nursing Expert Panel as "differences in the incidence, prevalence, mortality, and burden of diseases and other adverse health conditions that exist among specific populations groups in the United States" (Giger et al. 2007 p. 95), are the result of many factors, most of which may be out of our control. There is one area in which we as HCPs can and do make a difference, however, and that is culturally competent care in the hospital and clinic setting. This chapter assesses an organization's ability to embrace diversity, to provide culturally sensitive and competent healthcare to diverse populations, and to ensure a welcoming and respectful environment for all who walk through its doors: patients, community, and staff. It is more than patient care; it is about community outreach and a culturally diverse workforce. Each of these three areas is addressed, and each is pivotal in positive outcomes.

The journey begins with a vision and a belief that an institution that is culturally competent, sensitive, and aware can make a difference in health outcomes. It may seem like a daunting undertaking with questionable return on investment, but what if your organization became known as the premier healthcare institution in your city or your state? Results translate into patient satisfaction, high staff morale with low turnover, and good public relationships with the community.

Who we are . . . where we want to go

Having a vision, implementing the vision, and achieving the vision to become a culturally competent healthcare organization are a collaborative effort. Involvement of administrators, staff, and community is necessary. Administration must have a commitment to sustain the initiative and a dedication to provide funding and leadership. Staff acceptance is vital to the success of this initiative. Community participation offers insight into the needs of the population and helps to identify health issues. Thus, committees to facilitate this process need to include members from administration, staff, and community.

Who We Are . . . Where We Are Going, Figure 22-1, identifies current elements found in the organization (on the left) and elements that must be addressed (on the right) to make a successful transition to a culturally competent healthcare organization. It is a process that takes time, energy, good planning, and continued enthusiasm.

Who we are . . .	Where we are going . . .
Mission Statement	Information Sessions
Accreditation	Vision
Demographics	Focus groups
Policies/Procedures	Assessment Survey
Orientation Program	Goals & Objectives
Staff Evaluations	Budget & Timeline
Standards of Care & Practice	Revision of policies/procedures
Quality Assurance	Culltural competence criteria
Board of Directors	Educational Seminars

Figure 22-1: Who We Are . . . Where We Are Going

Information sessions

The process begins with information sessions for staff and community. This provides an overview of the proposed program: the purpose, timeline, benefits, and challenges. An opportunity to engage in discussion about the vision opens the door for staff to ask questions about the need for such a program and to understand the benefits to patient care. Community groups and leaders from churches, nonprofits, schools, and other organizations that use the health facility furnish the outside perspective of the health concerns and resources needed. The involvement of staff and community are vital to the process and key to the success of the program.

The Vision and The Mission

Reviewing Your Mission Statement
- Does it reflect the value of diversity found in the staff, patient, and community populations?
- Does it acknowledge cultural differences?
- Does it speak to providing a welcoming and respectful environment?
- Is it posted for all to see as they walk through the front door of the institution?
- Do the actions of staff and administration reflect the mission statement?

Creating or revising a mission statement to address cultural diversity is accomplished through dialogue with staff and community. It is a process, and when viewed as such, allows participants to hone in on the message and ultimately to take ownership. Those in the healthcare field sometimes prefer instant action over long-term discernment; however, when creating a culturally competent organization, additional time is going to make the end result more meaningful to all who participate in the process.

Reflective exercise: Creating a vision
1. *What is your vision of a culturally competent healthcare organization?*
2. *How does it address values of cultural diversity?*
3. *How does it address a welcoming environment?*
4. *Dignity for all who enter?*

Demographics – patient, staff and community

Demographics are changing all the time, albeit sometimes so subtly that we may not notice. Our patient and staff populations are not static. The community we served twenty years ago or even ten years ago may be vastly different from the clients or workforce today. If you work with a multiethnic staff and patient population, conflicts can occur because of varying cultural beliefs, values, biases, and practices. As you reflect on the following questions, think about the inconsistencies you discover . . . do you think they make a difference in patient outcomes, staff satisfaction, or community trust?

Reflective exercise: Do we reflect our community demographics?
1. *Administrators ~ do they reflect the community demographics?*
2. *Professional staff ~ the same question?*
3. *Ancillary staff ~ again the same question?*
4. *Patient demographics ~ if not reflective of community demographics could this lead to health disparities?*

Focus groups

Focus groups are a form of qualitative research in which people are asked about their perceptions, opinions, beliefs and attitudes toward a concept, idea, project, or product. Questions are designed to facilitate the discussions. The group is generally made up of six to ten people and a session lasts for approximately sixty to ninety minutes. The facilitator, selected and trained in group dynamics prior to the gathering, is responsible for explaining the purpose of the focus group, asking the pre-selected questions, encouraging discussion from all participants, and monitoring the flow. The information received is written down and/or recorded to ensure accuracy, compiled and submitted. These sessions can provide the opportunity for staff and community to verbalize their concerns, share ideas and develop a better understanding for the need to incorporate cultural sensitivity and competency into the vision of the organization. Listed below is a sample of the questions that could be asked during the session.

Sample questions for a focus group:
1. In what ways does the organization address cultural diversity?
2. What have been your experiences working with different cultural groups?
3. Do the departmental policies/procedures reflect the cultural beliefs, values, and practices of the patient population?
4. Do you think there is a need for cultural competency on the part of the staff? Administration?
5. What educational programs are in place for staff to meet the cultural needs of the patient population?

Assessment Surveys

In addition to the focus groups, written assessment surveys provide additional information that may not have been presented during the focus group session. Correlating both helps to identify areas that need to be addressed. There are several assessment tools available, so there is no need to "reinvent the wheel." The Health Resources Service Administration (HRSA), a department of the U.S. Department of Health and Human Services, furnishes one on their site: www.hrsa.gov/culturalcompetence. The assessment survey should include questions that address demographics, training needs, attitudes about cultural diversity, available resources and forms of communication.

Some of the questions that can be on a survey:
1. Are there printed materials or pictures that are reflective of the community population served?
2. Is written communication provided in the language of origin to those served?
3. Do videos and printed material for health education reflect the various cultures and languages of those being served?

Establish Goals and Objectives

Once the information from the assessment surveys and focus groups is compiled, it is then distributed to administration, staff, and community. Those who favor a transformation are probably eager to move on to the next step of establishing goals and objectives. Others, though, may not react with the same level of enthusiasm. If so, scheduling additional discussions to address these concerns and issues is helpful.

Identifying organization and departmental goals and objectives should be a collaborative process to include members from administration, staff, and community. Attention is given to formulation of goals and objectives that focus on the changes that need to occur with policy/procedures, orientation programs, evaluations, and education to ensure cultural competency. Ongoing communication using a variety of methods, such as e-mail, hospital and community newsletters, staff meetings, and informal conversations, assures that further concerns are addressed.

What we need to review . . .

Policies and procedures provide guidelines that ensure continuity throughout the organization. During this phase, a systematic review of policies and procedures is conducted to assess their relevance to providing culturally sensitive and competent services. The first question is: Does the value context, scope, purpose and policy align with the new vision statement? This process may seem daunting, as manuals are full to overflowing with policies and procedures, but individual departments can use the team approach to review and revise. Discussions at general meetings prior to finalizing helps to ensure credibility with staff. Here are some organizational and departmental policies and procedures that are relevant to cultural competency:

Organizational
- Admission policies
- Development of culture care standards and practice
- Working collaboratively with others to develop a cultural assessment tool.
- Hiring and recruiting practices

Departmental or Unit Based
- Visiting policies
- Admission Health Assessment
- Standards of Care and Practice

Orientation program . . . and cultural relevance

This program welcomes new employees and orients them to the organization's mission statement, core values, and policies and procedures, etc. Designing a program that includes components relevant to diversity ensures that the new hire understands the importance that culture plays in the delivery of care and interactions with colleagues. Review of policies, such as language in the workplace, education about cultural ways of dealing with conflict, and delivery of culturally sensitive healthcare, is beneficial.

> **Reflective exercise: Orienting to a new department . . . what to ask:**
> 1. *Does your departmental orientation program address cultural diversity?*
> 2. *Is there a policy addressing language spoken in the workplace?*
> 3. *Are cultural styles of communication and conflict resolution reviewed and discussed?*
> 4. *Is there discussion of the cultural values, beliefs, and health practices of your patient population?*
> 5. *Are Standards of Care and Practice reviewed?*
> 6. *What else needs to be added to the program?*

Evaluations

Annual evaluations are generally done as a collaborative process with input from the employee and the manager. It is a time to acknowledge accomplishments that have occurred over the past year and make suggestions for professional development. The decision to include cultural competence into the evaluation process raises the question of how to measure that concept. Cultural competence is not as tangible as arriving for work on time, attending staff meetings, or participating on a unit committee. Each department must define criteria specific to the service provided and population served. Staff from the unit can review and draw inspiration from the vision statement.

Here are some ways to address cultural competence in an evaluation:
- Attendance at cultural awareness education seminars
- Development of cultural standards of care and practice
- Work collaboration with other staff to develop a cultural health assessment tool
- Inservice presentation on an ethnic group representative of the department
- Chart documentation

Educational seminars

Cultural awareness education provides an opportunity for individuals in every area of the health organization (nurses, pharmacists, phlebotomists, nutritionists, housekeepers, and others) to acknowledge, appreciate, and respect their own cultural beliefs and values and to honor those who are different from themselves. These educational seminars should not be a cookbook approach to working with and caring for various ethnic groups, but rather a discovery of similarities and differences between the hospital staff and the patient – finding common ground.

A cultural awareness seminar must be informative, interactive, and motivating. Here are some components that should be part of a presentation:

- Demographics ~ patient population, staff, community, and state
- History and its influence on health decisions
- Stereotyping ~ Prejudice ~ Discrimination
- Barriers to Care ~ What gets in the way?
- Communication across cultures
- Health and folk care practices
- Family roles and responsibilities ~ Who makes decisions?
- Developing a plan of care that includes all the above

The Benefits and Challenges of Working with a Culturally Diverse Staff

The benefits may exceed the challenges when staff acknowledge the common ground that exists between cultural and ethnic groups. Workforce diversity seminars provide the opportunity for introspection and discussion which then leads to an acceptance of differences with patients and staff. It is in this process that we find common ground. The Purnell Model for Cultural Competence (Figure 22-2) is an excellent tool that can be used to develop a seminar for healthcare staff. This model, circular in design, highlights the global society, the community, the family, and the individual. The twelve domains are interactive and thus all must be considered. The journey is not static, but varies depending on a motivation to be culturally competent, interactions with staff and patients, experiences in the clinical arena, and educational opportunities. It begins with "unconsciously incompetent" and concludes with "unconsciously competent."

A workforce diversity seminar builds on previous cultural awareness education presentations and moves on to focus on components such as acculturation, communication, time management, conflict resolution, and individualistic/collectivistic approaches.

Acculturation . . . Over time

Acculturation occurs over time and is directly relational to socioeconomic and educational opportunities. For those immersed in the process of assimilation to a new country, each day brings challenges that require interpretation. For some employees who have recently arrived in the United States, this may seem like a never-ending activity that can cause anxiety and stress. It may be as slight as a questioning look from a colleague to an overt display of frustration following a misunderstanding. Being aware that this is a process and is not related to time spent in this country creates an understanding for the value of patience.

Communication . . . Understanding the Message

Communication is more than words. It is the unspoken message that is conveyed by tone of voice, gestures, and even silence. For those for whom English is a second language, the workplace may loom like foreign country, filled with misunderstanding. Continually translating during discussions, trying to pronounce words correctly, and conversing smoothly in a telephone

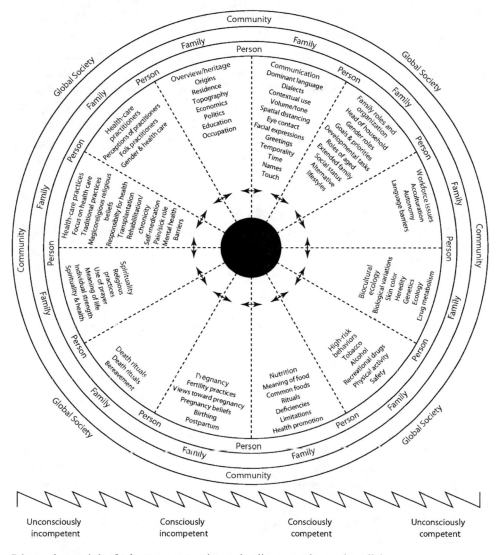

Unconsciously incompetent | Consciously incompetent | Consciously competent | Unconsciously competent

Primary characteristic of culture: age, generation, nationality, race, color, gender, religion

Secondary characteristics of culture: educational status, socioeconomic status, occupation, military status, political beliefs, urban versus rural residence, enclave identity, maritial status, parental status, physical characteristics, sexual orientation, gender issues, and reason for migration (sojoumer, immigrant, undocumented status)

Unconsciously incompetent: not being aware that one is lacking knowlege about another culture
Consciously competent: learning about the client's culture, verifying generalizations about the client's culture, and providing culturally specific interventions

Unconsciously competent: automatically providing culturally congruent care to clients of diverse cultures.

Figure 22-2: Purnell Model for Cultural Competence
Purnell Model for Cultural Competence.
Adapted with permission from Larry Purnell, Newark, Delaware.

conversation are daily challenges. Stress can add to the individual's inability to communicate effectively in English.

For the English-speaking staff, creating a relaxed atmosphere and repeating requests in a nonthreatening manner helps limited English-speaking staff understand the message. You may see the "nod and smile" response, which may translate into "I do not understand what you are saying, but to avoid embarrassment I'll say nothing." It is at these times that body language may speak louder than words. What are they not saying? Asking respectfully for understanding is an avenue to establishing rapport and trust.

Communication activities can include "real life events" submitted by staff. Building on the previous seminar in which participants received information about cultural differences, role play and/or group discussion can lead to a better understanding of the needs of the limited English person.

Time Management

Time is of the essence . . . or is it? For some in the dominant culture of the United States, "to be early is to be on time." This future orientation translates into the workplace message that organizing and prioritizing time to complete an assignment are very important. Meetings start on time, agenda items are set according to time, and punctuality by staff is an expectation.

Unfortunately, some staff members may view those who are always late as incompetent or uncaring. Both judgments perpetuate negative feelings and images that may lead to conflict. Time management for some cultural groups is in direct relationship to the "here and now." Patient or employee needs may supersede punctuality at a meeting. Tardiness is not done purposefully, but its value is relative. Discussion about the cultural values and beliefs about time orientation and how one manages his/her time is a good place to begin the dialogue. Discovering and accepting the varied approaches to time management helps staff/administrators to avoid future misunderstandings.

Conflict resolution

Resolution of conflict is approached from a variety of perspectives that are culturally learned. For some cultural groups, conflict is avoided, while others may use a third party to convey concerns because disrespecting those in authority may bring feelings of shame. For the individual in conflict, dignity can be preserved with silence as the third party representative pursues the resolution. The opposite is found in the dominant culture in the United States. Self reliance and assertiveness are valued. Seen on equal ground with others, an individual is expected to question decisions, and conflict is normal and natural. Resolution occurs, but probably not without some degree of tension, stress, anger, and possibly hurt feelings.

The opposite is found in the dominant culture in the United States. Self reliance and assertiveness are valued. Seen on equal ground with others, an individual is expected to question decisions, and conflict is normal and natural. Resolution occurs, but probably not without some degree of tension, stress, anger, and possibly hurt feelings.

Similar to previous activities, conflict resolution activities can include "real life" occurrences. They could involve a variety of situations: employee conflicts, management disagreements, or patient care conflicts. Present three scenarios and ask each member to write down how they would resolve the situation: avoid or confront. Then, as facilitator, present other options for discussion.

Individualistic and Collectivistic Approaches

Eighty percent of the world's cultures are collectivistic: the group is more important than the individual. Work is done in a collaborative spirit for the greater good of all. The value placed on harmony is in direct relation

INDIVIDUALISTIC	COLLECTIVISTIC
Autonomy valued	Harmony of group
Self-reliance	Relationship valued
Achievement oriented	Gentleness and cooperation
Directness valued	Indirectness valued
Responsibility for actions	Nonconfrontational resolution

Figure 22-3: Individualistic . . . Collectivistic

to hierarchy, which provides a structure to find one's place. Leaders are respected and followed. They are trusted to act in the best interest of the group and to make decisions on behalf of its members. That leaves twenty percent as individualistic: self-reliance and autonomy. It does promote and encourage voicing one's opinion about a situation and challenging another's perspective.

In what ways does your healthcare organization promote an individualistic approach, and where is collaboration encouraged? In a culturally diverse workforce, conflict can arise when leadership expects staff to work independently. Being open to other ways of working together helps to ensure a welcoming environment where all are respected.

Activities address the ways in which a department or a healthcare organization is individualistic and ways it promotes a collectivistic approach.

*   *   *   *

This chapter lays a foundation of cultural awareness and competence. The vision includes the voices of staff, administration, patients, and community. It is a process that includes willingness of all staff to actively participate. This collaborative effort, which takes time, money, and perseverance, helps to assure quality patient care, culturally competent staff, and the involvement of the community. Activities in the seminar can address the situation in which departments within the healthcare setting use an individualistic or collectivistic approach. This may enlighten staff and administrators to rethink the best approach in a given situation.

Resources

Andrews, M. M. (2008). Transcultural perspectives in nursing administration. In Andrews, M. M., Boyle, J. S. (Eds.). Transcultural Concepts in Nursing Care. (5th Ed.). New York: Lippincott Williams & Wilkins.

Campinha-Bacote, J. (2003). The process of cultural competence in the delivery of healthcare services: A culturally competent model of care. Cincinnati, OH: Transcultural C.A.R.E. Associates.

Gay, G. (2000). Culturally responsive teaching: Theory, research & practice. New York: Teachers College Press.

Georgetown University Center for Child and Human Development. National Center for Cultural Competence. www.georgetown.edu/research/guccdh/NCCC.

Giger, J. N., Davidhizar, R. E. (2008). Transcultural nursing: Assessment and intervention. (5th Ed.). St Louis, MO: Mosby/Elsevier.

Joint Commission on Accreditation of Healthcare Organizations. (2004). Standards, intents and examples for patient and family education and responsibilities.

Jones, P. S., Zhang, X. E., Siegl, K. J., Meleis, A. (2002). Caregiving between two cultures: An integrative experience. *Journal of Transcultural Nursing.* 13(3), 202-209.

Leininger, M. M. (1991). Culture care diversity and universality: A theory of nursing. New York: National League for Nursing Press.

Leininger, M. M., McFarland, M. R. (2002). Transcultural nursing: Concepts, theories, research and practice. (3rd Ed.). New York: McGraw-Hill.

Lipson, J. G., Dibble, S. O. (2005). Culture & Clinical Care. San Francisco CA: UCSF Nursing Press.

McGoldrick, M, Giordano, J., Garcia-Preto, N. (2005). *Ethnicity & Family Therapy.* (3rd Ed.). New York: Guilford Press

Menghini, K. G. (2005). Designing and evaluating parent educational materials. Advances in Neonatal Care. 5(5), 273-83.

Purnell, L. D., Paulanka, B. J. (2008). Transcultural Health Care: A Culturally Competent Approach. (3rd Ed.). Philadelphia, PA: F. A. Davis Company.

Sandoval, V. A., Adams, S. H. (2001). Subtle skills for building rapport using neuro-linguistic programming in the interview room. *FBI Law Enforcement Bulletin* 1-5.

Shusta, R. M., Levine, D. R., Wong, H. Z., Olson, A. T., Harris, P. R. (2008). *Multicultural Law Enforcement.* (4th Ed.). New Jersey: Pearson, Prentice Hall.

Spector, R.. (2009). Cultural diversity in health and illness. (7th Ed) New Jersey: Pearson/Prentice Hall.

Trumbull, E., Rothstein-Fisch, C. Greenfield, P. M., Quiroz. (2001). Bridging Cultures. New Jersey: Lawrence Erlbaum Associates.

U.S. Department of Health & Human Services. Health Resources and ServiceAdministration. www.hrsa.gov

Health Occupation Faculty . . . It All Begins Here

23

"I have lived in this country for over eleven years and I've always felt invisible. Since the first time I came to this college it's like I am not even in the classroom. I don't think my teachers even realize they are doing this.

– An Ethiopian nursing student

The faculty was silent. The students were silent. The hush in the room was penetrating. It took courage for her to speak up in front of her instructors. Her comment had more impact than any of us expected.

*   *   *   *

I was asked to present a seminar for health occupation faculty. The purpose of the presentation, titled Diversity & Healthcare: Translating it into Practice, was to provide faculty with the information and tools that would ensure students would graduate with skills to provide culturally competent healthcare. To my delight and surprise, the attendees included second year nursing students and peers. The Ethiopian nursing student validated all the research that says: faculty must be aware of their beliefs, values, and biases to ensure cultural competence in the curricula and clinical setting.

This chapter is written in memory of that encounter. It addresses nursing and faculty demographics, the barriers faced by minority students, accreditation requirements related to diversity, cultural assessment of faculty, and teaching strategies that include culturally diverse learning styles.

Demographics

Census demographics continue to indicate changes in the ethnic populations in the United States. Do students and faculty in health occupation programs reflect that change? Student demographics are changing at institutions of higher learning. However, the faculty demographics remain the same. The chart, Graduates from RN Programs (Figure 23-1), displays national statistics for students provided by the National League of Nursing (2000). Faculty demographics are from the American Association of Colleges of Nursing (2001).

Year	White	Black	Hispanic	Asian	American Indian
1984 (Students)	89.5%	4.5%	1.6%	3.0%	0.3%
2000 (Students)	77.2%	10.5	6.3%	5.1%	0.9%
2001 (Faculty)	87%	9%	1%	0.7%	1%

Figure 23-1: Graduates from RN Programs
Baccalaureate — Diploma — Associate Programs

Faculty continues to be predominately white, while student population is more diverse. It is a challenge to teach a culturally diverse student population; however, the rewards include opportunities to discover cultural ways of teaching that engage students who are eager to share information about their culture, their beliefs, and their health practices. It opens doors to understand possible perspectives that need to be considered in patient care.

Reflective exercise: Trends over time . . . the benefits and challenges
1. *What demographic changes have you seen in the student population?*
2. *In the faculty population?*
3. *What are the challenges of teaching in a culturally diverse student population?*
4. *How does faculty address those challenges?*
5. *What are the benefits?*

Barriers

Think about your experience as a nursing student. Did faculty reflect the ethnicity of the student population? Did students and faculty reflect the ethnicity of the patients? Did your curriculum include information about the cultural beliefs, values, and healthcare practices of diverse populations? Was faculty culturally sensitive to the learning needs of the diverse student body?

A study of health occupation faculty done by Yoder (1997) discovered that most of the educators did not consider student's cultural background to be an important factor in his or her education. Educators had low levels of cultural awareness and response to diverse student needs. The majority of faculty believed that all students, regardless of ethnicity, were basically the same. They were unable to identify barriers that culturally diverse students experienced.

From a student perspective, Janelle Gardner, PhD, (2005) discussed the need for a change in nursing education programs. The purpose of her study was to "document racial and ethnic minority student nurses' perspectives of their experience in predominately White nursing program" (p.156). Many times the minority students felt that their opinion was not valued by faculty or their white peers. Eight themes emerged.

Barriers Perceived by Minority Students
- Loneliness and isolation
- "Differentness"
- Absence of acknowledgment of individuality from teacher
- Peers' lack of understanding and knowledge about cultural differences
- Desiring support from teachers
- Coping with insensitivity and discrimination
- Determination to build a better future
- Overcoming obstacles

Gardner 2005

Each barrier can be part of the everyday experience of the minority student. Feeling lonely, isolated, and different creates additional stress that can impact learning in the classroom and clinical setting. The desire of the student to build a future for him or herself and family includes overcoming obstacles as well as coping with issues of prejudice and discrimination. While it may be uncomfortable for faculty to hear this information, recognition and support of the students' needs can lead to changes in the academic and clinical environment.

Promote Student Success	**Discourage** Student Success

Getting to know the student personally
Treating the student like an individual
  with wants, needs & desires
Encouraging
Approachable
Patient
Making the student feel comfortable
  around them
Caring
Showing compassion
Available
Organized
	Unapproachable
	Ignoring the student as a person
	Difficult to communicate with
	Lack of Understanding
	Disrespectful
	Intimidating
	Uncaring
	Disorganized
	Cold
	Not straightforward when answering
	  questions
	Not giving immediate feedback
	Inflexible Derogatory

Figure 23-2: Qualities of Nurse Educators that Promote & Discourage Success
Source: Used with permission: J. Gardner TCNJ 2005 16 p.159

Accreditation and Student Learning Outcomes

There are six regional accreditation bodies in the United States. They are responsible for all schools from elementary through college. Accreditation serves to ensure quality and adherence to academic standards, and it determines eligibility for federal and state financial aid programs.

The Commission on Collegiate Nursing Education offers accreditation of baccalaureate and master's nursing programs, and clinical nursing doctorate programs. Standards related to the mission statement and student learning outcomes are used to assess an academic institution. Another accrediting body is the American Commission for Community and Junior College (Western Region). Here are the standards reflecting the learning needs of the diverse student population.

Standard II: Student Learning Programs and Services

- The institution identifies and seeks to meet the varied educational needs of its students through programs consistent with their educational preparation and the **diversity, demographics and economy of its community**
- The institution uses delivery modes and teaching methodologies that **reflect the diverse needs and learning styles of its students**
- The institution validates its effectiveness in measuring student learning and **minimizes test biases**

Learning styles vary from culture to culture. Those coming from within the United States are familiar with the western style of an individualistic approach to learning and testing. Those from foreign countries may subscribe to a collectivistic and verbal approach using essays to test the student's knowledge. A successful educational program draws from both. Being attentive to these differences and incorporating them guarantees success in reaching students and meeting their educational needs.

Reflective exercise: Student learning outcomes
1. *Who accredits your institution?*
2. *What are the student learning outcomes specific to your department?*
3. *How are cultural learning styles addressed in the development of curricula and testing?*
4. *Do you see any biases?*

Assessing Cultural Competency . . .

Assessment of faculty's cultural awareness, sensitivity, and competency opens doors to changes in curricula and student interaction. Not all faculty believe there is a need for such an evaluation. While many have worked with diverse student populations and believe they are culturally astute, research indicates otherwise as cited in the works of Yoder and Granelle.

There are several tools available to assess cultural competence. Camphina-Bacote's tool, Inventory for Assessing the Professional Cultural Competence (IAPCC), determines the cultural awareness and competence of the individual on a scale ranging from culturally incompetent to culturally proficient. It is initially administered to determine where a faculty member is on the continuum. This process, repeated after educational and experiential opportunities have taken place, is a good indicator of movement toward competency. Doing a departmental cultural assessment can serve as a talking point at staff meetings and helps to identify the need for further diversity education.

A second assessment tool is the Intercultural Development Inventory, a tool developed by Drs. Bennett and Hammer. It measures five orientations toward cultural difference based on Dr. Bennett's Developmental Model of Intercultural Sensitivity. The assessment reveals the way individuals construe their social world in terms of dealing with cultural differences between themselves and people from other social and cultural groups. Measured on a continuum, it begins with the ethnocentric approach of denial/defense and moves toward the ethnorelative stage of acceptance and adaptation. The results provide cultural assessment for the individual and/or the organization and help to identify future training and education needs.

As a prelude to completing any assessment, it is essential for there to be opportunities for faculty to discuss the need. Addressing this sensitive subject is difficult for many, but the end results help to assure more positive outcomes for faculty and students.

> **Reflective exercise: Self and Department Cultural Assessment**
> 1. *Have you ever completed a cultural self awareness assessment tool?*
> 2. *What were the results . . . Were they what you expected?*
> 3. *Did you find it helpful?*
> 4. *Were you involved in the decision-making process to do this exercise?*
> 5. *Did new programs . . . new teaching strategies . . . better communication emerge?*

Where to next . . . Teaching Strategies and Cultural Awareness

Can one exist without the other? Teaching styles used by faculty are diverse. What is your style? How do you incorporate cultural awareness into your curricula? In her research on faculty and cultural awareness, Marian Yoder EdD, RN, identifies five styles of teaching.

<u>Patterns of Teaching</u>

1. **Generic** ~ ethnicity not considered important in the educational process; all students are the same
2. **Culturally non-tolerant** ~ not willing to tolerate cultural differences; no accommodation to students' cultural beliefs and ways of learning

3. **Mainstreaming** ~ strategies directed at repatterning students' behavior to meet expectations of dominant society; attempt at repatterning cultural ways

4. **Struggling** ~ increased awareness of cultural differences, struggling to adapt strategies to respond to cultural needs; faculty acknowledged need to be more culturally competent in order to interact with diverse student populations

5. **Bridging** ~ encouraged students to maintain ethnic identity and modified strategies to meet the cultural needs of the students

Marian Yoder 1997 p. 317

Reflective exercise: Five Teaching Patterns
1. *Which pattern is most reflective of your teaching style?*
2. *Which style intrigues you?*
3. *What resources are available to enrich your cultural teaching strategies?*

In the classroom . . .

Culturally aware and competent faculty recognizes and accepts that values, beliefs, and cultural ways of learning influence outcomes. Yoder (2001) posits that there are four conditions that influence faculty's cultural awareness level: lived experience, participation in sensitivity sessions, experience interacting with diverse students, and commitment to equity. Here are some strategies used by Bridging Educators.

Effective Strategies of Bridging Educators
- Incorporating students' cultural knowledge
- Preserving cultural or ethnic identity
- Providing successful ethnic role models
- Facilitating negotiation barriers

Three Additional Teaching Strategies . . .

Three teaching methods are reviewed in this section: Interactive activities, a course based on the constructivist theory, and curricula using the Giger-Davidhizar Model for Transcultural Assessment and Intervention. Each provides an opportunity to gain understanding of the cultural beliefs, values, and practices of various ethnic populations.

The American Association of Nursing Education together with experts in the field of cultural competence developed an educational program for baccalaureate nursing programs. The Tool Kit of Resources for Cultural Competence Education for Baccalaureate Nurses contains content and strategies faculty to use in the classroom and clinical areas This toolkit, for undergraduate and graduate nursing programs, is available at the AACN site at www.aacn.nche.edu/education/cultural

Strategies such as role play, story telling and group activities offer creative learning venues. As individuals, we learn through a combination of feeling, watching, thinking, and doing. Effective learning opportunities can include individualistic (individual) and collectivistic (group) activities. The individual approach relies solely on the student's ability to learn, while group activities offer familiarity for those who prefer a collaborative or team approach (Mexican, Filipino, Chinese, and more). Given that information, a class comprised of culturally diverse students should include a variety of methods to reach the learning objectives.

Storytelling, found in cultures with an oral tradition (such as Native American and Hawaiian, Chinese, and Hmong), is an effective way to share information. This method allows individuals or a group to provide classmates with stories about their culture, views about health and illness, spiritual beliefs, and traditional folk practices. Storytelling opens us up to new concepts and thoughts. It helps to hone our listening skills, thus we are able to gain more information from our patients.

Case presentations offer an excellent way to talk about the benefits and challenges of caring for patients from various cultural groups. This group approach enables students to work collaboratively to gather information and to present it to the class. The presentation can focus on specific or a variety of aspects of an ethnic group. These can include such concepts as the patient/family beliefs about healers and healing methods; family roles and responsibilities and decision making; or beliefs about death and dying.

Outside speakers can provide insights into cultural ways of living and healing. At a recent conference titled Latina Woman: Health & Wellness, three curanderas (Mexican healers) spoke about their healing practices and their relationship with the community. For many of us it was a first time experience and expanded our view of healers.

Periodicals, such as the *Journal of Transcultural Nursing*, provide current research, and educational and clinical practice articles that enrich the world of faculty and students. There are many periodicals and websites available that offer information about cultural diversity and healthcare. The National Center for Cultural Competence at Georgetown University (www. georgetown.edu) offers curriculum development as well as assessment tools.

Reflective exercise: in the classroom setting
1. *What are some of the resources you currently use?*
2. *What teaching strategies have you used in the classroom?*
3. *Are they effective?*
4. *Does faculty work collaboratively to develop these programs?*
5. *Are they part of your overall mission statement . . . goals/objectives . . . of the department?*

A Constructivist Approach in the Classroom

The curricula based on the constructivist theory posits that learning is an ongoing process in which the person "constructs" and "reconstructs" information in order to learn. Hunter (2008) applied this approach when teaching cultural care for diverse populations to her nursing students. Her nursing students were encouraged to share their stories. They discovered common ground with peers. This method allows students to bring their experiences into the conversation in the classroom and clinical setting. This course was developed in conjunction with the four constructs of "cultural awareness," "cultural knowledge," "cultural skill," and "cultural encounters" found in Camphina-Bacote's model (2003). Cultural awareness highlights the need for awareness of one's prejudices and biases toward other ethnic, religious, gender, or generational groups. Cultural knowledge stresses the importance of having a solid base of information about different cultures, including their values, beliefs, and healthcare practices. Cultural skill asks students to use a cultural assessment tool to interview a person from a cultural group that is different from their own. Finally, cultural encounters suggest that multiple interactions with various ethnic groups promote awareness, understanding, and knowledge that leads to cultural competence in the clinical setting. In addition to the cognitive and experiential assignments, there are readings and discussions. Discussions allow the students to express their perspectives and to glean insights and ideas from each other.

Giger-Davidhizar Transcultural Nursing Assessment

In response to the need for tools to guide the HCP in identifying the beliefs, values, and health practices of various ethnic groups, Joyce Giger, EdD, RN, and Ruth Davidhizar, DNS, RN, developed a cultural assessment model (Figure 23-3 & 23-4). Using this model in the clinical setting helps to ensure that a student gathers all aspects of the patient's culture: communication, time, space, social organization, environmental control, and biological variations. Giger and Davidhizar provide a questionnaire that can assist the student in this interviewing process.

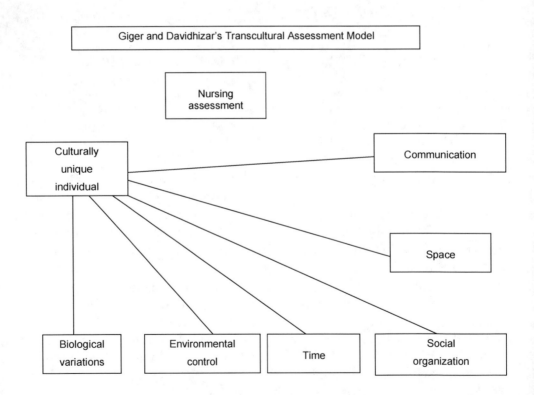

Figure 23-3: Giger and Davidhizar's
Transcultural Assessment Model
Giger, J.N., Davidhizar, R.E. (2008). Transcultural Nursing:
Assessment and Intervention. (5th Ed.) St. Louis, MO: Mosby/Elsevier
Used with permission

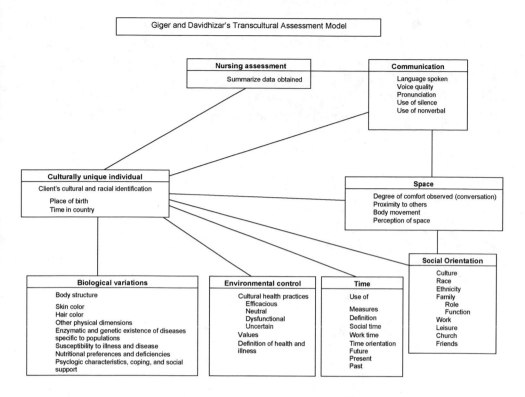

| Giger and Davidhizar's Transcultural Assessment Model |

**Figure 23-4: Giger and Davidhizar's
Transcultural Assessment Model**

Giger, J.N., Davidhizar, R.E. (2008). Transcultural Nursing:
Assessment and Intervention. (5th Ed.) St. Louis, MO: Mosby/Elsevier
Used with permission

Doing a cultural assessment on oneself and then on a peer builds the student's confidence to use it in the clinical setting. Faculty can facilitate a group discussion following this exercise to help students determine what they learned personally and how they are different from their peers. The goal is to find common ground.

*   *   *   *

The students are the future HCPs. Faculty can make a difference by providing an understanding of culture and the influence that it has on health. There are a variety of approaches and strategies to instill cultural awareness, knowledge, skills, and competence; however, faculty must be culturally astute and competent first. Together, culturally competent faculty and students address the reality of changing ethnic populations and their healthcare needs.

Resources

American Commission for Community and Junior College (Western Region). Standards: Student Learning Programs and Services. Retrieved on November 3, 2009, from http://www.accjc.org

American Association of Colleges of Nursing. (2001). Issue bulletin: Effective strategies for increasing diversity in nursing programs. Retrieved July 9, 2007, from http://www.ancc/nche.edu/publications/issues

Andrews, M. M., Boyle, J. S. (2008). Transcultural concepts in nursing care. (5th Ed.).New York: Lippincott Williams & Wilkins.

Calvillo, E., Clark, L., Ballantyne, J. E., Pacquiao, D., Purnell, L. D., Villarruel, A. M. (2009). Cultural Competency in Baccalaureate Nursing Education. *Journal of Transcultural Nursing.* (20)2, 137-145.

Campinha-Bacote, J. (2003). The process of cultural competence in the delivery of healthcare services: A culturally competent model of care. Cincinnati, OH: Transcultural C.A.R.E. Associates.

Choi, L. L. (2005). Literature review: Issues surrounding educational of English-as-a-second language (ESL) nursing students. *Journal of Transcultural Nursing.* (16)3, 263-268.

Coffman, J. M., Rosenoff, E., Grumbach, K. (2001). Racial/ethnic disparities in nursing. *Health Affairs.* (20)3, 263-272.

Gardner, J. (2005). Barriers influencing the success of racial and ethnic minority students in nursing programs. *Journal of Transcultural Nursing.* (16)2, 155-162.

Giger, J. N., Davidhizar, R. E. (2008). Transcultural nursing: Assessment and intervention. (5th Ed.). St Louis, MO: Mosby/Elsevier.

Gilchrist, K. L., Rector, C. (2007). Can you keep them? Strategies to attract and retain nursing students from diverse populations: Best practices in nursing education. *Journal of Transcultual Nursing.* (18)3, 277-285.

Hassounch-Phillips, D., Beckett, A. (2003). An education in racism. *Journal of Nursing Education.* (42)6, 258-265.

Hunter, J. L. (2008). Applying constructivism to nursing education in cultural competence. *Journal of Transcultural Nursing.* (19)4, 354-362.

Kovner, C., Fairchild, S., Jacobson, L. (2006). Nurse educators 2006: A report of the faculty census survey of RN and graduate programs. Retrieved March 6, 2010, from www.nln.org\research

Labun, E. (2002). The Red River college model: Enhancing success for Native Canadian and other nursing students from disenfranchised groups. *Journal of Transcultural Nursing.* (13)4, 311-317.

Leininger, M. M. (1999). Faculty limit students' study of transcultural nursing: A critical issue. *Journal of Transcultural Nursing*. (10)3. 258-259.

Leininger, M. M. (1991). Culture care diversity and universality: A theory of nursing. New York: National League for Nursing Press.

Leininger, M. M., McFarland, M. R. (2002). Transcultural nursing: Concepts, theories, research and practice. (3rd Ed.). New York: McGraw-Hill.

Peters, M. (2000). Does constructivist epistemology have a place in nursing education. *Journal of Nursing Education*. (39)4, 166-172.

Powell-Kennedy, H., Fisher, L., Fontaine, D., Martin-Holland, J. Evaluating diversity in Nursing Education. *Journal of Transcultural Nursing*. (19)4, 363-370.

Purnell, L. D., Paulanka, B. J. (2008). Transcultural Health Care: A Culturally Competent Approach. (3rd Ed.). Philadelphia, PA: F. A. Davis Company.

Rew, L., Becker, H., Cookston, J., Khosropour, S., Martinez, S. (2003). Measuring cultural awareness in nursing students. *Journal of Nursing Education*. (42)6, 249-256.

Selig, S., Tropiano, E., Greene-Moton, E. (2006). Teaching cultural competence to reduce health disparities. *Health Promotion Practice*. (7)3, 247S-255S.

Shearer, R., Davidhizar, R. (2003). Using role play to develop cultural competence. *Educational Innovations*. (42)6, 273-276.

Sowers-Hoag, K. M., Sandau-Beckler, P. (1996). Educating for cultural competence in the generalist curriculum. *Journal of Multicultural Social Work*. (4)3, 37-57.

Spector, R.. (2009). Cultural diversity in health and illness. (7th Ed) New Jersey: Pearson/Prentice Hall.

Stolder, M. E., Hydo, S. K., Zorn, C. R., Bottoms, M. S. (2007). Fire, wind, earth and water: Raising the education threshold through teacher self-awareness. *Journal of Transcultural Nursing*. (18)3, 265-270.

Yoder, M. (1997). The consequences of generic approach to teaching nursing in a multicultural world. *Journal of Nursing Education*. 35, 315-321.

Yoder, M. (2001). The bridging approach: Effective strategies for teaching ethnically diverse nursing students. *Journal of Transcultural Nursing*. 12, 319-325.

Glossary

Acculturation: adaption of a person from one cultural group to another; may occur in stages over a long period of time

Acupuncture: Chinese method of restoration of Yin/Yang through the use of inserting needles into meridians to remove blockage to qi.

Allopathic: health beliefs based on scientific model; technology, prescribed meds; immunization

Amor propio: save face and maintain self esteem (Filipino American)

Amulet: an object that is thought to offer protection against illness or evil spirits; tying string to wrist (Hmong American), attaching safety pin to clothing (pregnant Mexican woman)

Apocopation: style of communication when the end of one word is a vowel as is the beginning of the word in a phrase. Example: ¿Como esta usted?" may sound like "¿Comoestausted?"

Ayb: shame caused to a Muslim woman by discussing a female health issue with a male doctor

Bible: the holy book of Christianity

Biomedicine: an approach to health and illness; based on scientific information; cause and effect; also known as western medicine

Boat people: second wave of immigrants coming from Vietnam in the mid 1970s

Class: people having the same social or economic status

Coining: a method healing in which a coin is placed on the skin; when dark ecchymotic spots appear it means the treatment is working

Complicated grief: a sense of loss that includes a person being frozen or stuck in a state of chronic mourning and unable to make adaptations to life

Constructivist theory: used in the academic setting to build on students' experience and current knowledge and to introduce new information

Cuarentena: forty-day period following childbirth (Mexican American)

Curandero: healer in the Mexican culture

Culture: values, beliefs, attitudes transmitted from one generation to another, often tacitly; each influence the way one sees the world

Cultural awareness: understanding one's own beliefs and values; recognizing the similarities and differences with other groups

Cultural competence: self awareness coupled with the knowledge of the cultural beliefs and health practices of other groups, acknowledging differences and finding common ground; providing health care that is within the cultural context of the patient.

Cultural humility: ongoing process of self reflection and self critique of interactions with others

Cultural imposition: imposing one's cultural views and biases on another

Cupping: applying small heated cuplike forms to skin that cause suction and leave ecchymotic spots; remedy for joint and muscle pain and to remove excess wind

Dab: malevolent spirits found in the Hmong health beliefs

Dau: word for pain in the Vietnamese language

Discrimination: prejudicial behavior or treatment toward individuals or groups of people that involves restricting members of one group from opportunities that are available to other groups

Ethnicity: groups who have different experiences and backgrounds ~ customs, social factors, religion

Ethnocentrism: belief that one (group) is superior to another

Exercise bulimia: an intensive exercise regime used compulsively to control weight

Hajib: head covering for women (Islam American)

Halal: requirement by Muslims that meat be properly slaughtered and prepared

Health care disparity: differences in the incidence, prevalence, mortality, and other adverse health conditions that exist among specific groups

Hevrah-Kadisha (Chevra Kadisha): a holy society that prepares the body for burial (Judaism)

Hilot: healer in the Filipino culture

Hiya: avoid shame (Filipino American)

Holistic: viewing the individual within the context of mind, body, spirit, and community

Homeopathic: a natural approach to healing

Immigrant: a person who voluntarily came to a host country

In sha Allah: God willing

Kaddish: prayer that praises God and affirms one's faith (Judaism)

Kahuna: Hawaiian healer

Kosher: diet that does not include pig products or shellfish; meat and milk are not eaten together.

Locus of control: internal is when the person believes he or she has control over the body and environment; external is the belief that anything that happens is a result of fate, luck, or chance.

Magioreligious: folk medicine taking into consideration religion and folk beliefs

Medicine wheel: a symbol used in the Native American culture to show wholeness by balance of mental, emotional, physical, and spiritual components.

Meridians: sites where qi flow crosses; acupuncture needles are inserted at these sites to restore flow

Moxibustion: Chinese method of healing through use of heat

Naturalistic: an approach to health and illness; belief that illness is caused by imbalance in the body ~ hot/cold, Yin/Yang, wind

Neeb: healing spirit in the Hmong belief system

Pakikisama: maintain smooth relationships (Filipino American)

Personalistic: an approach to health and illness; belief that illness is caused by intervention of a supernatural being (diety/god), nonhuman (ancestor, ghost), or human (witch, sorcerer)

Personalismo: maintain a respectful relationship

Prayer warriors: women of the African American church community who offer prayers on behalf of those who are in need

Qi (chi): a term for energy found in all living things

Qur'an: holy book of Islam; furnishes guidelines for all aspects of life

Race: a group with biological similarities

Racism: belief that one's race to superior to another

Refugee: sponsored by the government; comes to the country as the result of religious or political persecution; war; genocide

Reiki: healing method; reduces stress and restores health by transferring energy from the practitioner's hand to the client's body

Religion: an organized system of beliefs; offers guidelines for practices and assurance gained through prayer and worship

Shaman: healer

Simpatico: maintain smooth relationships; avoid conflict

Spirituality: a personal approach to finding life's purpose, finding meaning to life

Sweat lodge: a structure that is used for healing and purification; hot rocks are placed strategically; herbs such as sweetgrass, sage, and cedar are used (Native American)

Talisman: blessed religious object that offers protection from illness and evil spirits

Torah: holy book of Judaism

Txiv Neg: Hmong healer

Yin & Yang: Chinese concept of the understanding of balance in the universe; Yin (female) and Yang (male) co-exist to ensure the complementary balance

Yoga: a physical exercise and meditative activity that helps with balance

About the Author

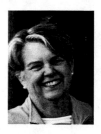

Beth Lincoln, MSN, RN

Beth Lincoln, MSN, RN, received her Masters in Nursing and Women's and Family Health, with Nurse Practitioner certification from University of California, San Francisco. As a Nurse Practitioner, she has provided clinical healthcare and professional education for a diverse population, and in *Reflections from Common Ground . . . Cultural Awareness in Healthcare*, she illustrates some of the situations in which cultural diversity may affect healthcare, including methods and means for health professionals to gain multi-cultural competence. Ms. Lincoln is a Certified Transcultural Nurse, credentialed by the Transcultural Nursing Society, where she currently serves as the International President. Additionally, she is an Administrator of the Intercultural Development Inventory, as certified by The Intercultural Communication Institute. Ms. Lincoln presents extensively, sharing her broad understanding and inspiring others to strive for cultural competence in providing sensitive and effective health care.

Ms. Lincoln is the founder of Celemonde!, a cultural awareness educator for healthcare, scholastic and business institutions and individuals. A pathway to reflection and discovery, the Celmonde! way engages diverse professionals in a new dialogue to better appreciate how cultural issues can influence their effectiveness and decisions and create conflict in their workplace. By creating greater cultural awareness, we can open the door to common goals and better understanding. Ms. Lincoln encourages each of us to celebrate every individual as a unique opportunity to share the colorful history we all represent and the rich fabric we can become by weaving our diverse strands together.

To discover more about the Celemonde! way contact Ms. Lincoln at
www.celemonde.com